Correlative Neuroanatomy

THE ANATOMICAL BASES of Some Common Neurological Deficits

Duane E. Haines, Ph.D.
Professor and Chairman
Department of Anatomy
The University of Mississippi Medical Center
Jackson

Urban & Schwarzenberg
Baltimore-Munich

Urban & Schwarzenberg, Inc.
7 E. Redwood Street
Baltimore, Maryland 21202
USA

Urban & Schwarzenberg
Landwehrstrasse 61
D-8000 Munchen 2
West Germany

Library of Congress Cataloging in Publication Data

Haines, Duane E.
Correlative neuroanatomy.

Bibliography: p.
Includes index.
1. Neuroanatomy. 2. Nervous system—Diseases—Diagnosis.
3. Syndromes. I. Title. [DNLM: 1. Nervous System—anatomy & histology. 2. Nervous System—pathology. WL 101 H153c]
QM451.H17 1985 611'.8 85-3281
ISBN 0-8067-0881-6

Printed in the United States of America
Second Printing - September 1985
Third Printing - July 1987
Fourth Printing - January 1990

ISBN 0-8067-0881-6 Baltimore

ISBN 3-541-70881-6 Munich

CONTENTS

Foreword by Ludwig Gutmann, M.D....v

Preface....vi

Acknowledgments....vii

Introduction....1

Chapter 1: The Spinal Cord....2

Chapter 2: The Medulla Oblongata....22

Chapter 3: The Pons....38

Chapter 4: The Midbrain....54

Chapter 5: The Cerebellum....66

Chapter 6: The Diencephalon, Visual System, Basal Ganglia, Internal Capsule, and Cerebral Cortex....74

Sources and Selected References....96

Index....99

FOREWORD

Duane Haines and his colleagues have, over the past many years, made the neuroanatomy course for our first year medical students at West Virginia University an interesting one. They have done so both by their enthusiasm for the subject and their ability to provide meaningful clinical correlations emphasizing the significance of important anatomical structures and pathways.

This volume is an outgrowth of these efforts. It presents the neuroanatomical structures and pathways in a graphic and easy to understand fashion and relates them to a series of important neurological syndromes. The clinical features of each syndrome are neatly correlated with the neuroanatomical abnormalities. An appreciation of these correlations is essential if one wishes to localize the clinical findings presented by each example in the correct area of the nervous system and fully understand why certain signs and symptoms occur. As every neurological clinician knows, this process of localization is the first step in making a correct diagnosis of what is the actual underlying lesion when one is faced with a given set of signs and symptoms referrable to the nervous system.

Medical students and residents in neurology and neurosurgery will find this volume extremely useful in their understanding of the neuroanatomical substrate for the various important syndromes illustrated. At the same time, it adds considerable spice to their learning and/or reviewing the more important neuroanatomical structures and pathways about which they need to know.

Ludwig Gutmann, M. D.
Professor and Chairman
Department of Anatomy
The University of Mississippi Medical Center
Jackson

PREFACE

The ultimate goal in modern neurobiology courses is to provide a factual and conceptual framework for understanding how the nervous system functions. To this end, examples of neurologic problems, in the form of lesions and their accompanying deficits, are frequently used to emphasize particular points.

To fully understand the losses resulting from a lesion one must be able to visualize the origin, course, and termination site of fibers which pass through the damaged region. Many neurobiology students (as well as others who later in their careers must review neural connections) experience difficulty visualizing (or remembering) tracts or pathways in their entirety. Although a lesion may be small and located in one area it usually produces wide spread deficits. These are seen as various types of dysfunctions, e.g., alternating losses versus unilateral losses, many of which are seen at some distance from the injury site. The value of using example lesions in learning/reviewing human neurobiology is to develop a concept of how the deficits correlate with the trajectory of the interrupted fibers. Where are these fibers coming from, what information are they carrying, where do they decussate (if they do), and where do they terminate? If one can answer this series of questions in relation to a given lesion, one will more clearly understand the accompanying deficits.

The goal of Correlative Neuroanatomy is to provide a framework for visualizing pathways as functional entities in three dimensions. The approach is to describe briefly a lesion (many commonly seen, some used for their instructive value), correlate the deficits with their appropriate structures, and review the trajectory of fibers interrupted by the injury. Emphasis is placed on showing not only what structures may be involved at the lesion site, but where the fibers are coming from, where they cross the midline, and where they terminate. It is not the intent of this book to teach clinical aspects of neuroscience. The clinical examples are used to illustrate, teach, and review the functional organization of connections within the central nervous system. The example lesions are from current human neurobiology texts and the clinical literature.

Since all possible examples can not be included, each chapter is designed to provide instruction, review, and self-study. Example lesions which the reader has the option to analyze, and blank master drawings on which lesions and corresponding pathways of the reader's (or instructors) choice can be planned are included in each chapter.

Effective use of this book presumes a certain amount of previous knowledge or on-going instruction. Consequently, it is viewed as a companion resource to the variety of textbooks and atlases currently available. Its design may be useful to students in their first exposure to human neurobiology in medical, dental, graduate and a variety of allied health curricula, as well as to anyone seeking a succinct correlative review. An effort has been made to develop illustrations that are informative and helpful at many different levels of study.

There are three features of this book which, when considered collectively, make its approach unique. First, it correlates information (deficit-structure-tract organization) in a visual/review format. Second, all fibers shown are printed in red. If the reader wishes to add additional pathways to those offered this can be conveniently done in the same, or another, color. Third, the self-study component in each chapter provides the reader with the opportunity to expand significantly his or her knowledge.

I readily acknowledge that I have probably left out someone's 'favorite case'. For this and other foibles that may have crept in, I am solely responsible. I welcome comments, corrections, and suggestions from my basic science and clinical colleagues, as well as from students, interns, and residents.

Duane E. Haines
Morgantown
January, 1985

ACKNOWLEDGMENTS

The author is deeply indebted to a variety of individuals who have greatly contributed to the completion of this work. My colleagues in the Department of Anatomy have been very supportive. I especially appreciate the help of Dr. Jim Culberson. He reviewed, in detail, all sections of this work and offered many helpful suggestions and comments; his input has unquestionably improved the quality of the final product. I have also solicited suggestions from Drs. Tom Sowa and Richard Frederickson (Anatomy) and from teaching colleagues in the Department of Physiology (Drs. Paul Brown, W. Gladfelter and R. Millecchia). Dr. Ludwig Gutmann, Professor and Chairman of Neurology and a teaching colleague for many years in our Medical Neurobiology course, also gave generously of his time. He reviewed the entire work, offered many important suggestions and comments, and graciously consented to write the Foreword. I sincerely appreciate his interest in this project.

Since this work is designed with the medical student in mind, I have also received help from this sector. Two individuals in particular, Michael Rubenstein (Class of 1985) and Richard DeAngelis (Class of 1987), have reviewed all parts of the work and made suggestions which have been incorporated in the hope the other students will benefit. Other members of the medical classes of 1985, 1986, and 1987 have also provided important suggestions. I am also indebted to my Chairman, Dr. Robert McCuskey, for providing an atmosphere which encourages academic endeavors.

This work would never have been completed without the talents of Mr. Clyde Koon, Ms. Lydia Moon and Ms. Lois E. Williams. Mr. Koon, Biomedical Photographer, did all the photography. His skill and ability to get the very best out of our drawings resulted in photographs of the highest quality. Ms. Moon made exact ink copies of the original pencil renderings of the author. Her patience with this task and with the tedious job of labeling all the figures is gratefully acknowledged. Ms. Williams typed all portions of the manuscript. She not only did an excellent job, but put up with the author through numerous changes and corrections. I am also indebted to Ms. Anne Carr and Mr. Cary Johnson for their untiring cooperation. To Dr. Claude Sherrill, Director of Biomedical Photography, I express my thanks for his interest in this project.

A special note of thanks is due the personnel of Urban & Schwarzenberg. Mr. Norman Och answered numerous questions, provided many important suggestions, and supervised the design and production of the finished product. To Ms. Nan Curtis Tyler, Editor, Mr. Charles W. Mitchell, Associate Editor, and Mr. Braxton Mitchell, President, I express my appreciation for their numerous suggestions and comments and for their interest in bringing this work to fruition.

D.E.H.

INTRODUCTION

Correlative Neuroanatomy is designed to help the reader correlate the deficits resulting from a given lesion with the trajectory of fibers passing through the damaged area. A three dimensional visual base for understanding the relationship between the deficit and the structures involved is provided so that the transition from lesion to involved tracts is as expeditious as possible. Each set of facing pages addresses a specific problem. The illustration on the left page shows the position and extent of a lesion as an area of oblique lines; principle structures are also labeled. The deficits seen as a result of the lesion are correlated with the appropriate structure in tabular format immediately below the illustration. The same base illustration is shown on the right page, the extent of the lesion again indicated, and the trajectory through the lesion of those fibers responsible for the deficits are superimposed on this drawing in red. Below this illustration the locations of cells of origin and the sites of their terminations are summarized for each tract shown. The transition from lesion and associated deficits (left page) to the trajectory of the main tracts involved (right page) can be easily made without searching through other sections of the book.

To further expedite the learning and/or review process, self-study components are built into each chapter; these are provided in two forms. First, immediately following sets of lesion illustrations for which the pathways have been outlined, are sample lesions which involve specific structures for which the deficits and corresponding connections are not provided. To assess his or her understanding of structural-functional relationships the reader may indicate the corresponding deficits (left page) and trace the trajectory of fibers and indicate the locations of their cells of origin and sites of termination (right page). The design of the second self-study feature was based on the fact that all possible lesions could not be included. This second feature could be appropriately called "Make Your Own Lesion." At the end of each chapter, a blank master drawing is provided on which lesions of any size, shape and extent can be constructed. Space is provided for listing deficits and their corresponding structures. The blank drawing on the facing page can be used to outline the trajectory of pathways involved or to trace projections to and from cranial nerve nuclei. Readers may also wish to tabulate information on the origin and termination of whatever tracts they choose. In this way the reader or instructor is not restricted to the examples shown, but can tailor the book to the specific needs of a wide range of teaching/learning/reviewing situations.

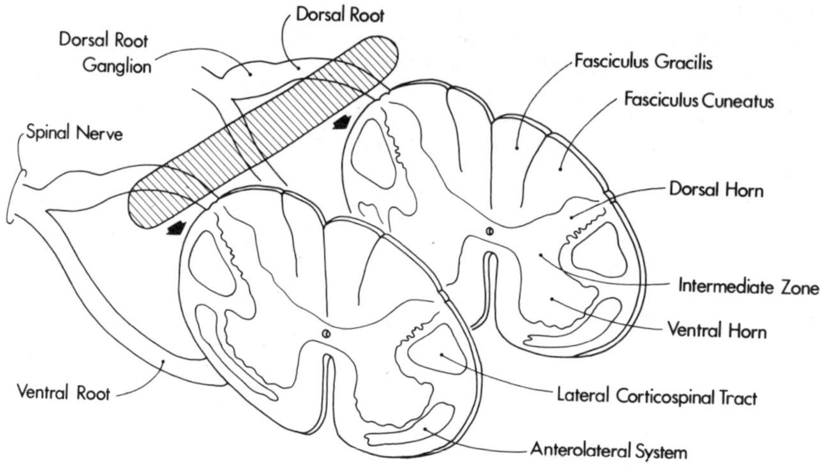

Fig. 1-1. TUMOR INVOLVING THE DORSAL ROOTS AT C_6-C_7: The most common types of extramedullary tumors found inside the dura are meningiomas and neurofibromas. They may involve dorsal and/or ventral roots and cause mild to severe compression of the spinal cord. The example shown here involves dorsal roots and represents a complete block of the C_6-C_7 roots with mild compression of the dorsolateral aspect of the spinal cord.

DEFICIT	ASSOCIATED STRUCTURE
A. Ipsilateral loss of pain, temperature, and touch sensation on lateral aspect of arm, forearm, and on thumb, diminution of position and vibratory sense on thumb and at the elbow, hyporeflexia of triceps and biceps	A. Dorsal roots at C_6 and C_7
B. Ipsilateral hyperreflexia (patellar, Achilles), Babinski sign, weakness in arm, forearm, and leg	B. Compression (arrows) of lateral corticospinal tract

COMMENT: Initial compression of the dorsal roots may cause radicular pain (or root pain) accompanied by paresthesias (numbness, tingling or pricking sensations). As the pressure on the roots increase there is eventually a complete loss of all sensations over portions of the C_6 and C_7 dermatomes. Severe compression of the cord may result in some components of a Brown-Sequard syndrome.

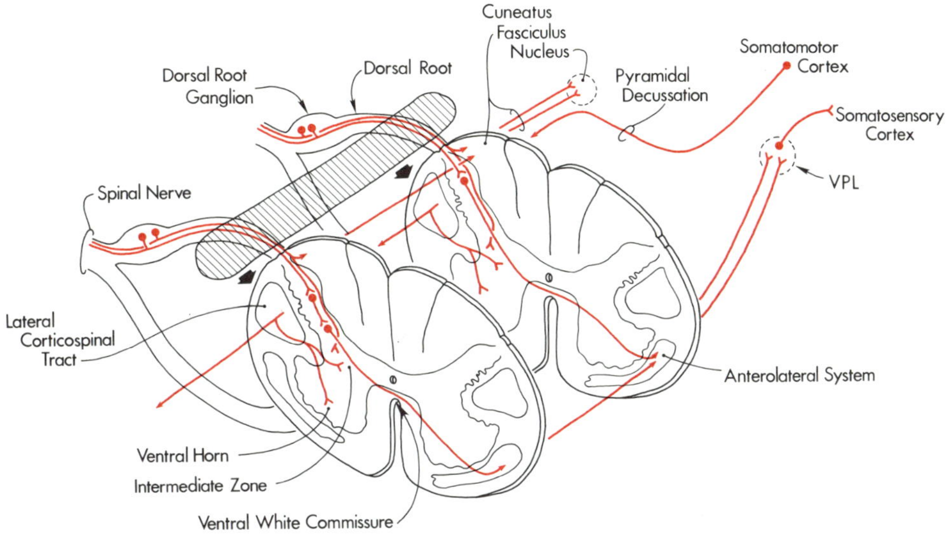

Fig. 1-2. Trajectory of fibers responsible for the symptoms seen when a tumor compresses the dorsal roots at C_6-C_7 and puts some pressure on the spinal cord.

TRACT/FIBERS	RELATIONSHIP TO LESION	
	CELLS OF ORIGIN	TERMINATION
A. Dorsal roots at C_6-C_7	Ipsilateral dorsal root ganglia at these levels	Ipsilateral dorsal horn laminae I-VI (exteroceptive fibers) and ipsilateral nucleus cuneatus (proprioceptive fibers)
B. Corticospinal fibers	Contralateral somatomotor cortex	Ipsilateral ventral horn and intermediate zone below this level

COMMENT: Due to the extramedullary location of the tumor, sensory losses are primarily seen in the C_6-C_7 peripheral distribution. Sensory information from other regions of the body relayed via intramedullary pathways, such as the dorsal columns and anterolateral system, may be intact, especially if the tumor is small.

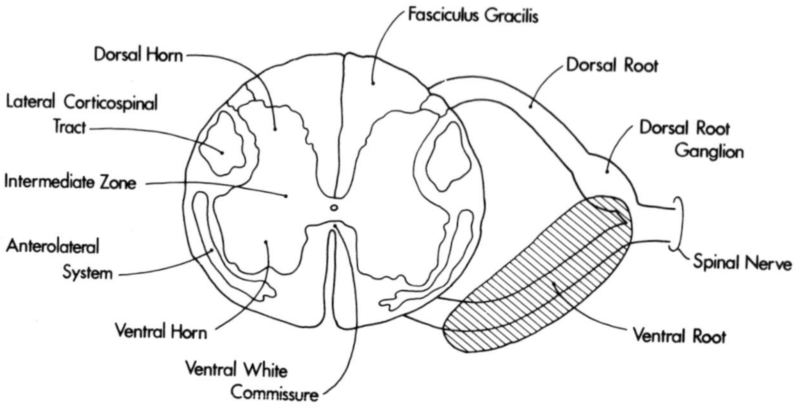

Fig. 1-3. HERNIATED NUCLEUS PULPOSUS INTO THE L_4-L_5 INTERSPACE: At the L_4-L_5 interspace a herniated disc will involve the L_5 ventral root and may extend into the intervertebral foramen compressing the L_5 dorsal root and/or ganglion. The nucleus may displace the posterior longitudinal ligament without passing through it (protruded disc) or may pass through the ligament (extruded disc).

DEFICIT	ASSOCIATED STRUCTURE
A. Ipsilateral hypesthesia and/or pain referred to anterior and lateral aspects of the leg and to the large, second and third toes	A. Compression of the dorsal root and/ or ganglion at the L_5 intervertebral space
B. Less obvious motor deficits, some weakness of the ipsilateral anterior and posterior tibial muscles	B. Compression of the L_5 ventral root

COMMENT: Herniation of the nucleus pulposus may be caused by a variety of actions which place abnormal strain on the vertebral column. The onset may be sudden with extreme pain or gradual with a growing sense of numbness or pain. Movement may either momentarily relieve or exacerbate the pain. Motor deficits are a less common sign; they may be documented using electromyography. The primary, and most consistent, complaint is varying degrees of pain.

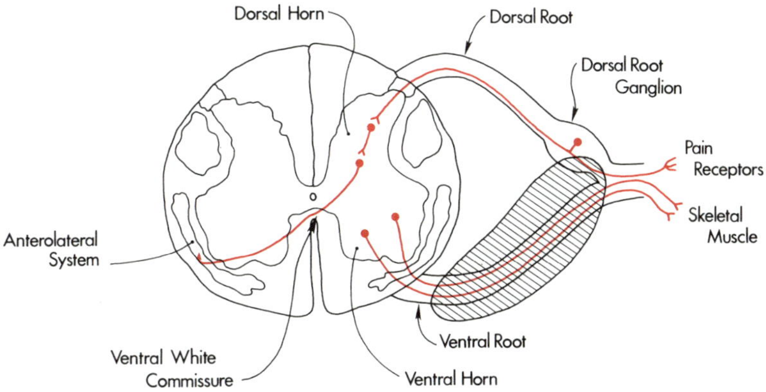

Fig. 1-4. Trajectory of fibers and locations of cells responsible for the symptoms seen in compression of the L_5 roots (and ganglion) subsequent to a herniated nucleus pulposus.

TRACT/FIBERS	RELATIONSHIP TO LESION: CELLS OF ORIGIN	RELATIONSHIP TO LESION: TERMINATION
A. Dorsal root and/or ganglion	Cells in the ipsilateral dorsal root ganglion	Ipsilateral dorsal horn laminae I-VI
B. Ventral root	Ipsilateral ventral horn	Ipsilateral somatic musculature served by the involved root

COMMENTS: Compression of a single ventral root will produce minimal motor deficits which may be only detected using electromyography. A herniated disc which compromises two adjacent ventral roots may produce a noticeable flaccid paralysis (lower motor neuron lesion) and eventual atrophy of the muscles served.

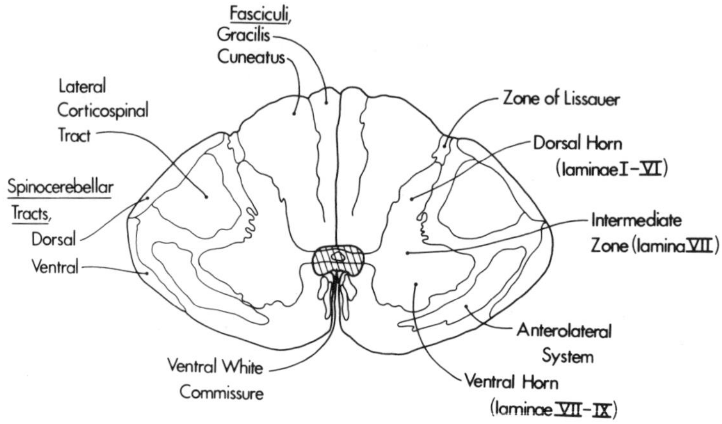

Fig. 1-5. **SYRINGOMYELIA AT C_4 - C_8:** This is a cavitation of central areas of the spinal cord that may spread into adjacent areas of gray and white matter. The cavity is frequently surrounded by an area of gliosis. This may be caused by small vascular hemorrhages or occlusions, traumatic insults, infections, neoplasms (astrocytomas), or congenital malformations (vascular). The example shown here is in an early stage.

DEFICIT	ASSOCIATED STRUCTURE
A. Bilateral loss of pain and temperature sensation on lateral aspect of arms, forearms, and on thumbs, index fingers and middle fingers	A. Ventral white commissure
B. None	B. Lamina X of spinal gray

COMMENT: Syringomyelia is sometimes referred to as hydrosyringomyelia, syringohydromyelia, myelosyringosis or Morvans disease. One characteristic of syringomyelia is that it frequently has a significant longitudinal extent within the spinal cord and may involve decussating fibers of the ventral white commissure over considerable distances. The loss of pain and temperature sensation is uniquely bilateral due to the damage to the decussating fibers.

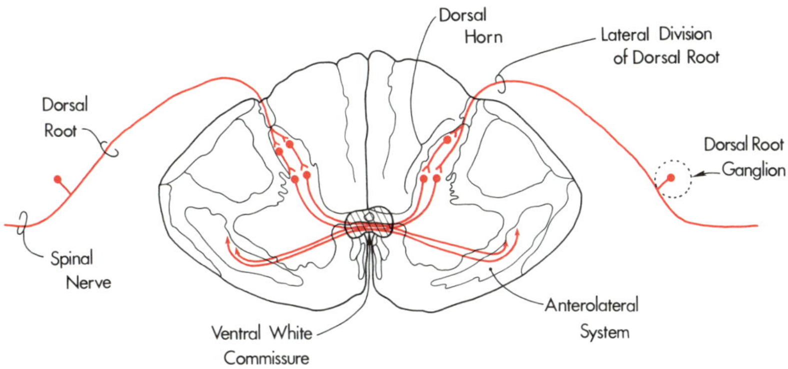

Fig. 1-6. Trajectory of fibers responsible for the symptoms seen in a syringomyelia at C_4 - C_8.

	RELATIONSHIP TO LESION	
TRACT/FIBERS	CELLS OF ORIGIN	TERMINATION
A. Ventral white commissure	Bilateral laminae I-VI of the dorsal horn	Bilateral VPL of thalamus

COMMENT: The bilateral segmental loss of pain and temperature is due to damage of crossing fibers in the ventral white commissure. Progressive enlargement of this lesion may involve surrounding structures (see Fig. 1-7,1-8), such as the ventral horns, various portions of the dorsal column system, and, in extreme cases, the long ascending fibers of the anterolateral system.

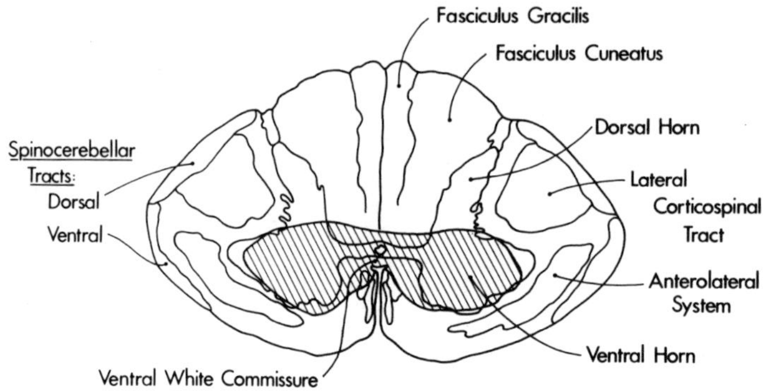

Fig. 1-7. **SYRINGOMYELIA FROM C_3-T_4.** The cavitation in syringomyelia may extend into adjacent areas of the cord. A large cavitation may be the result of a traumatic insult alone or it may result from trauma to a pre-existing vascular malformation. The example shown here involves central cord areas and the ventral horns.

DEFICIT	ASSOCIATED STRUCTURE
A. Bilateral loss of pain and temperature sensation on the shoulder, arm, forearm, hand, back (upper third of scapula) and chest (down to just above the nipple)	A. Ventral white commissure from C_3-T_4
B. Bilateral weakness or flaccid paralysis of muscles of shoulder, arm, forearm, and hand	B. Ventral horn from C_3-T_4

COMMENT: A more extensive cavitation that would involve lateral corticospinal tracts, anterolateral system fibers, or dorsal column fibers would result in appropriate deficits. In addition, the cavitation may extend more into one half of the cord than into the other producing an asymmetry of signs.

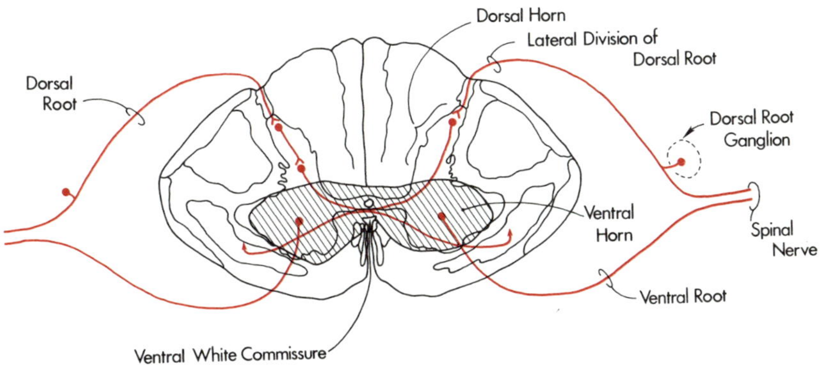

Fig. 1-8. Trajectory of fibers and locations of cells responsible for the symptoms seen in a large syringomyelia extending from C_3-T_4.

	RELATIONSHIP TO LESION	
TRACT/FIBERS	CELLS OF ORIGIN	TERMINATION
A. Ventral white commissure	Bilateral dorsal horn laminae I-VI	Bilateral VPL nucleus of thalamus
B. Ventral horns	Cell bodies of the ventral horns, bilateral involvement	Bilateral somatic musculature of shoulder, arm and hand

COMMENT: A small part of the dorsal columns is shown within the lesion. Such minimal involvement would not precipitate any obvious loss of function. More extensive intrusion of the lesion into the dorsal columns would result in a bilateral loss (assuming symmetry of the lesion) of position and vibratory sense. Paresthesias or a loss of pain and temperature sensation over portions of the body below the T_4 level may occur bilaterally if ascending fibers within the anterolateral system (spinothalamic fibers) are involved.

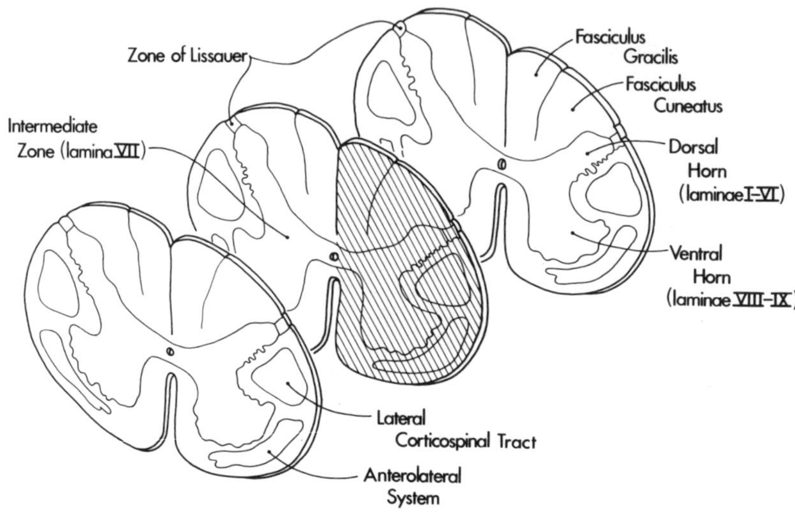

Fig. 1-9. BROWN-SÉQUARD SYNDROME AT C4: Hemisection of the spinal cord. Although not frequently seen in its most classic form, this may result from a traumatic insult or be seen as a sequel to pressure exerted on the cord from an extramedullary tumor.

DEFICIT	ASSOCIATED STRUCTURE
A. Ipsilateral loss of position and vibratory sense and discrimination touch below level of lesion	A. Fasciculi gracilis and cuneatus and and dorsolateral funiculus
B. Contralateral loss of pain and temperature sensations beginning about one segment below the lesion	B. Anterolateral system (spinothalamic fibers)
C. Ipsilateral spastic hemiplegia of arm, forearm, and leg	C. Lateral corticospinal fibers (also reticulospinal, rubrospinal, vestibulospinal)
D. Ipsilateral constriction of pupil, bilateral diminution (or loss) of sweating, reflex bladder	D. Descending multisynaptic pathways through the reticular formation to autonomic spinal centers (not shown)

COMMENT: The spastic paralysis of the arm and leg are presumably related to interruption of descending extrapyramidal fibers (i.e., rubrospinal, vestibulospinal, reticulospinal as main examples). Various portions of the overall Brown-Séquard syndrome are frequently seen in a variety of spinal cord injuries.

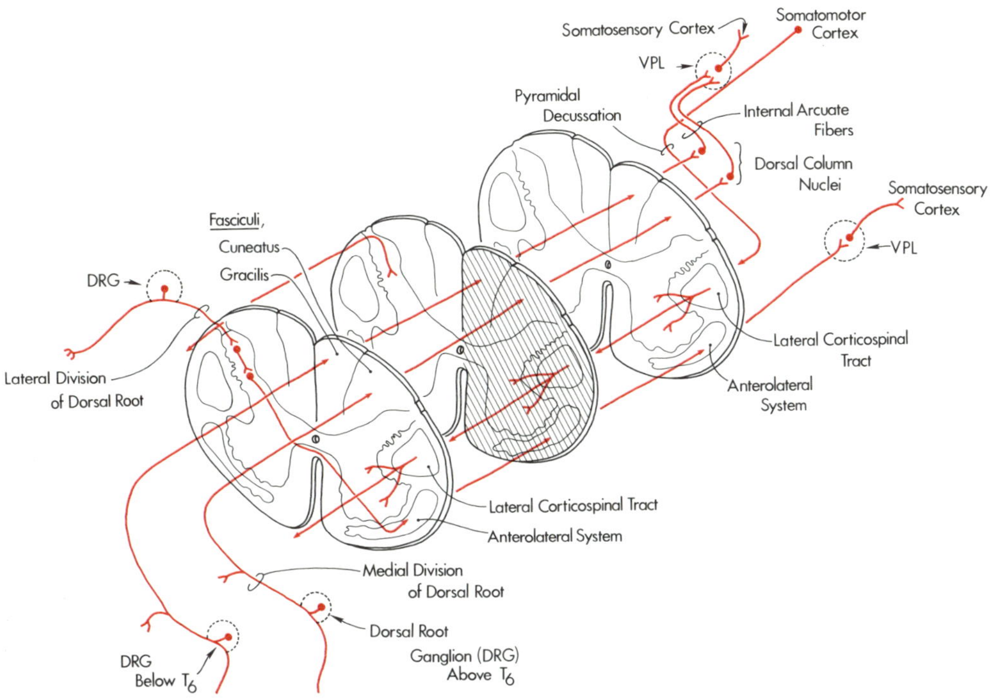

Fig. 1-10. Trajectory of principal fibers responsible for the symptoms seen in a Brown-Séquard syndrome at C_4.

	RELATIONSHIP TO LESION	
TRACT/FIBERS	CELLS OF ORIGIN	TERMINATION
A. Fasciculus gracilis	Ipsilateral dorsal root ganglia below T_6	Ipsilateral gracile nucleus
Fasciculus cuneatus	Ipsilateral dorsal root ganglia above T_6	Ipsilateral cuneate nucleus
Dorsolateral funiculus (not shown)	Ipsilateral lamina IV-V of spinal gray	Ipsilateral lateral cervical nucleus
B. Anterolateral system	Contralateral lamina I-IV of spinal gray	Ipsilateral VPL of thalamus
C. Lateral corticospinal	Contralateral somatomotor cortex	Ipsilateral spinal gray
Rubrospinal fibers (not shown)	Contralateral red nucleus	Ipsilateral spinal gray
Reticulospinal and vestibulospinal fibers (not shown)	Bilateral reticular and ipsilateral vestibular nuclei	Ipsilateral spinal gray

COMMENT: Ascending fibers in the dorsolateral funiculus originate mainly from cells in the nucleus proprius and terminate in the ipsilateral lateral cervical nucleus. Cells of the lateral cervical nucleus project to the contralateral VPL via the medial lemniscus.

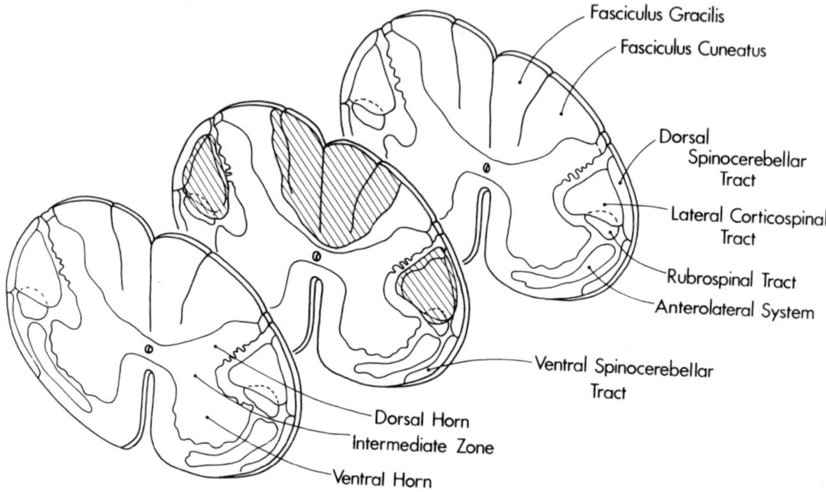

Fig. 1-11. SUBACUTE COMBINED DEGENERATION OF THE SPINAL CORD: This is a neurological condition seen in pernicious anemia. The lack of a gastric intrinsic factor results in a malabsorption of vitamin B_{12}. The result is a bilateral subacute degeneration of the spinal cord, peripheral nerves and to a lesser extent the cerebral hemispheres. The areas of the spinal cord most frequently involved are the dorsal columns and the dorsal part of the lateral funiculus. The example shown here is representative of low cervical and upper thoracic levels.

DEFICIT	ASSOCIATED STRUCTURE
A. Bilateral loss (or impairment) of position and vibratory sense in legs, some ataxia	A. Dorsal columns (primarily the fasciculus gracilis)
B. Bilateral spastic weakness of legs, increased Achilles and patellar reflexes, Babinski sign	B. Corticospinal tracts, descending extrapyramidal fibers

COMMENT: Involvement of the dorsal columns may also include the fibers of the cuneate fasciculus. This, in combination with damage at mid or high cervical levels, would precipitate a bilateral loss of position and vibratory sense in the upper extremity. Likewise a bilateral weakness of the upper extremity (corticospinal fibers) would result from cord damage at mid to high cervical levels. Paresthesias (numbness, tingling sensations), indicating involvement of peripheral nerves, may also be present. As the disease progresses the arms are affected, but not as severely as the legs. Mental deterioration, presumably related to involvement of the cerebral hemispheres, is seen in many cases. The expected spasticity may disappear, or not even occur depending on the degree of peripheral nerve involvement. The spastic paralysis of the lower extremities is related to damage to descending extrapyramidal fibers (rubrospinal and reticulospinal).

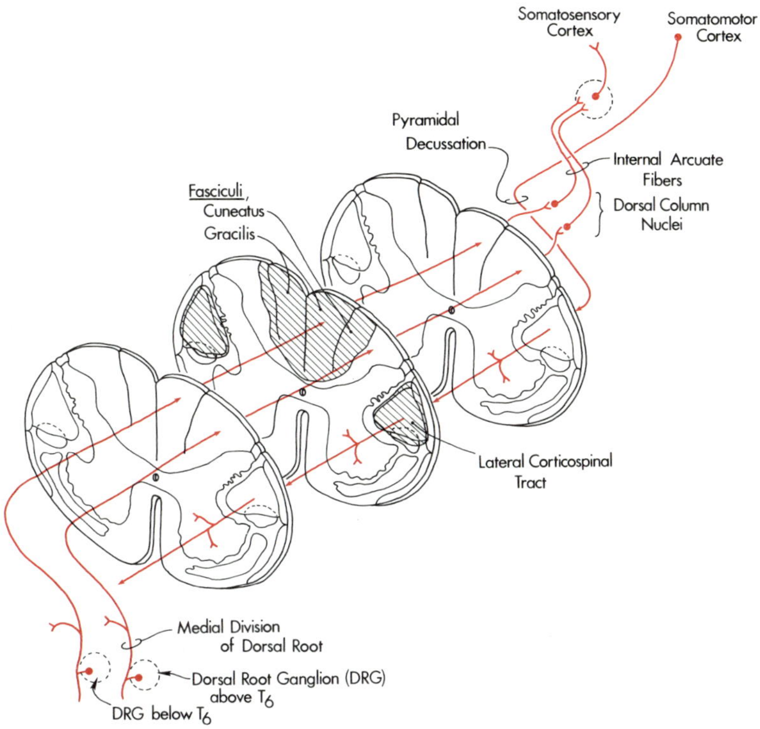

Fig. 1-12. Trajectory of fibers responsible for the symptoms seen in subacute combined degeneration of the spinal cord at low cervical and upper thoracic levels.

	RELATIONSHIP TO LESION	
TRACT/FIBERS	CELLS OF ORIGIN	TERMINATION
A. Fasiculus gracilis	Ipsilateral dorsal root ganglia below T_6	Ipsilateral nucleus gracilis in medulla oblongata
B. Lateral corticospinal tract	Contralateral somatomotor cortex	Ipsilateral spinal gray at and below level of lesion

COMMENT: Although the dorsal columns (usually the fasciculus gracilis) and lateral corticospinal tract are most frequently involved in subacute combined degeneration of the spinal cord, degenerative changes may also be seen in other areas of the cord. Paresthesias of the extremities may be related to involvement of the anterolateral system (spinothalamic fibers) or, more likely, to degenerative changes of peripheral nerves. The trajectory of fibers through the anterolateral system is shown in Fig. 1-10. Descending extrapyramidal fibers are not shown on this illustration.

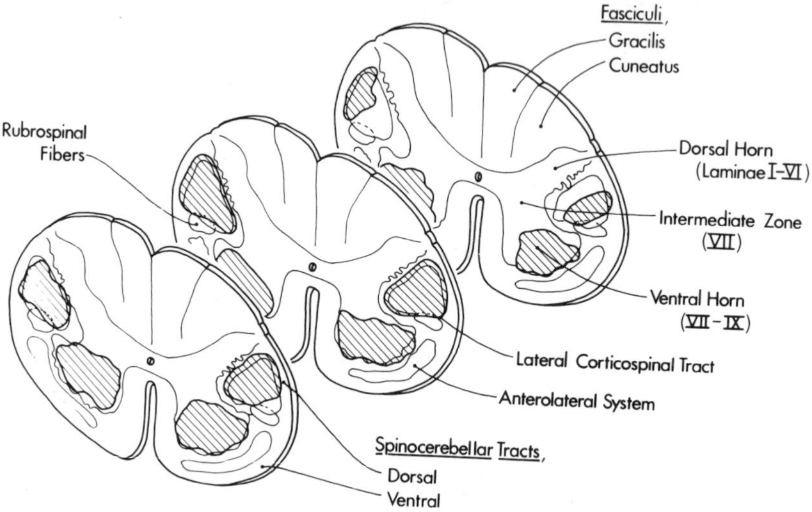

Fig. 1-13. **AMYOTROPHIC LATERAL SCLEROSIS:** Although a disease of unknown etiology viral and genetic origins have been suggested. In the sporadic form there is neuronal loss in the somatomotor cortex, in some motor nuclei of cranial nerves, and in the ventral horn of the spinal cord. In the inherited form, cells of Clarke's nucleus and fibers of the dorsal columns and spinocerebellar tracts degenerate. The example shown here is of the sporadic form at cervical levels.

DEFICIT	ASSOCIATED STRUCTURE
A. Bilateral weakness, fasciculations, and atrophy of muscles of arm, forearm and hand	A. Ventral horn
B. Bilateral weakness and spasticity of the legs, increased tendon reflexes, Babinski sign	B. Lateral corticospinal tracts and descending extrapyramidal fibers

COMMENT: Degenerative changes may take place at restricted cord levels (e.g., only cervical or lumbar, etc.) or throughout many levels. In the bulbar form degenerative changes are most frequently seen in motor nuclei of the trigeminal, facial and hypoglossal nerves and in the nucleus ambiguus. The losses would correlate with the nuclei involved.

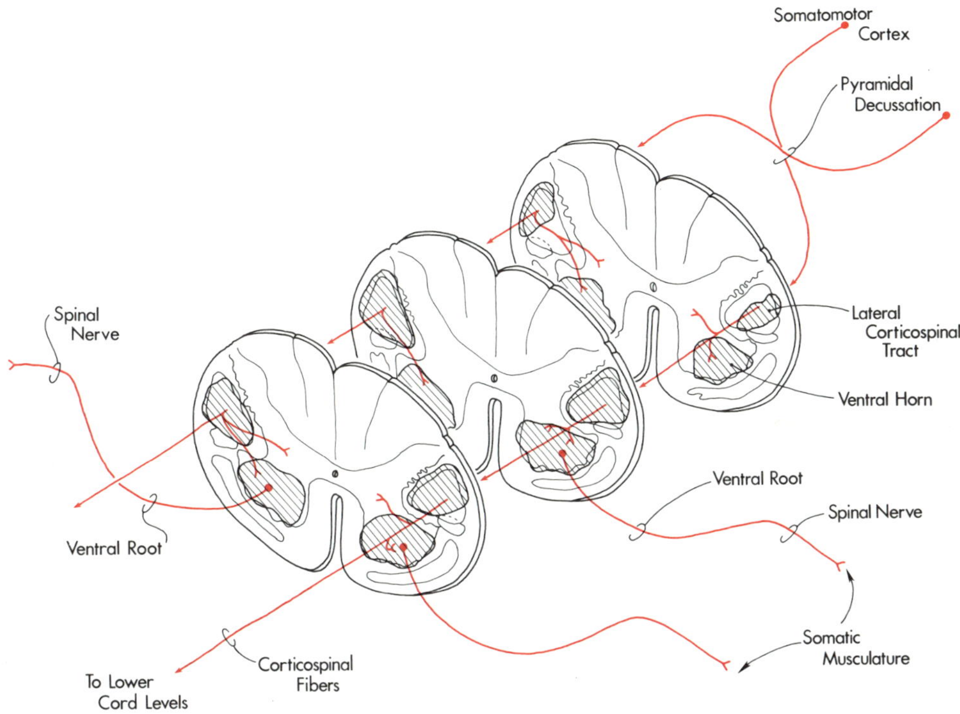

Fig. 1-14. Trajectory of fibers responsible for the symptoms seen in amyotrophic lateral sclerosis at cervical levels.

TRACT/FIBERS	RELATIONSHIP TO LESION	
	CELLS OF ORIGIN	TERMINATION
A. Axons from ventral horn cells	Ventral horn cells	Ipsilateral somatic musculature of the upper extremity
B. Lateral corticospinal fibers	Contralateral somatomotor cortex	Ipsilateral ventral horn and intermediate zone at and below the level of the lesion

COMMENT: Descending extrapyramidal fibers (reticulospinal, vestibulospinal, rubrospinal) may be partially involved and would explain the spasticity that is seen.

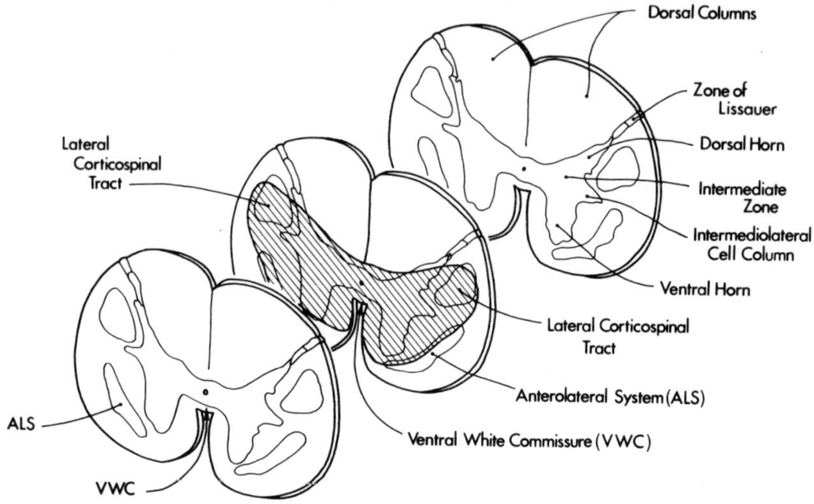

Fig. 1-15. ACUTE ANTERIOR THORACIC CORD INJURY AT T_5-T_7: This is the result of traumatic insult to the vertebral column with resultant displacement of the vertebrae and compression of the cord and/or its blood supply.

DEFICIT	ASSOCIATED STRUCTURE
A. Bilateral complete loss of pain and temperature sensation on thorax just below nipples	A. Ventral white commissure at T_5 to T_7; may also include T_4 and T_8 levels
B. Bilateral partial loss (or paresthesias) of pain and temperature below level of lesion	B. Anterolateral system (long ascending spinothalamic fibers)
C. Bilateral spastic paresis of legs, reflexes may initially be hypoactive, becoming hyperactive with time, Babinski sign	C. Lateral corticospinal tract and descending extrapyramidal fibers

COMMENT: In this example preservation of the dorsal columns indicate that the symptoms may result from compromise of the blood supply. Severe dislocation or fracture of the vertebrae would probably directly damage the cord and signs of dorsal column involvement would be seen. If the cord is crushed or severed the deficits are permanent. Mild compression of the cord or a temporary interruption of its blood supply may produce transient deficits with a partial and/or complete return of function with time.

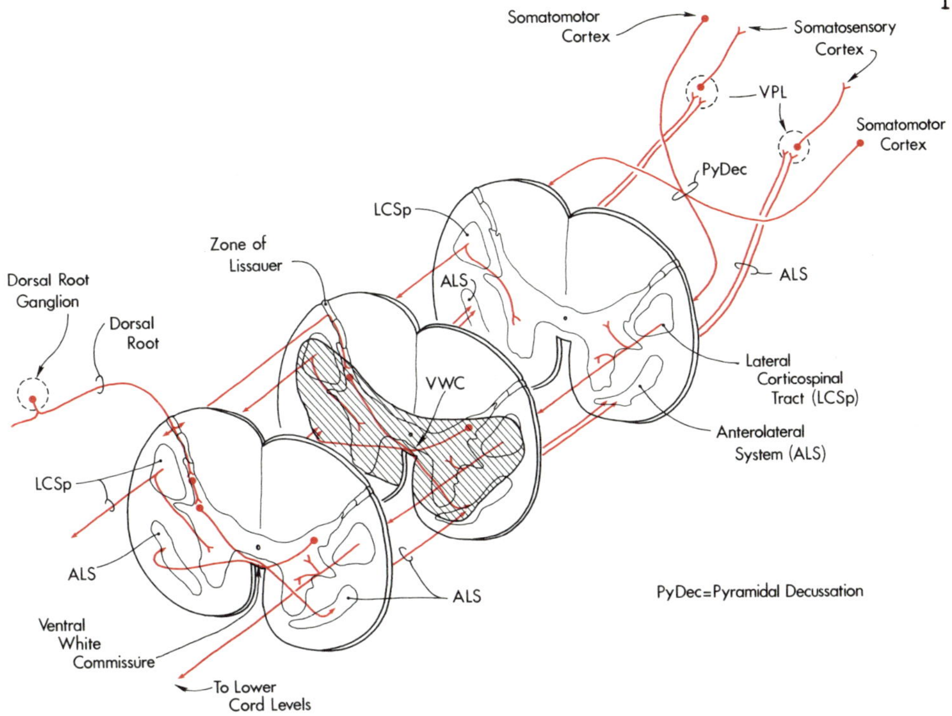

Fig. 1-16. Trajectory of fibers responsible for the symptoms seen in an acute thoracic cord injury at T_5-T_7.

	RELATIONSHIP TO LESION	
TRACT/FIBERS	CELLS OF ORIGIN	TERMINATION
A. Ventral white commissure (crossing fibers)	Bilateral dorsal horn lamina I-VI	Bilateral VPL of thalamus via the anterolateral system
B. Anterolateral system (ascending fibers)	Contralateral dorsal horn lamina I-VI	Ipsilateral VPL of thalamus
C. Lateral corticospinal tract	Contralateral somatomotor cortex	Ipsilateral ventral horn and intermediate zone at and below lesion level

COMMENT: The partial loss of pain and temperature sensation may be seen as an irregular spotty pattern over the lower trunk and legs. This is due to the fact that only medial parts of the fibers comprising the anterolateral system are involved in the area of the lesion.

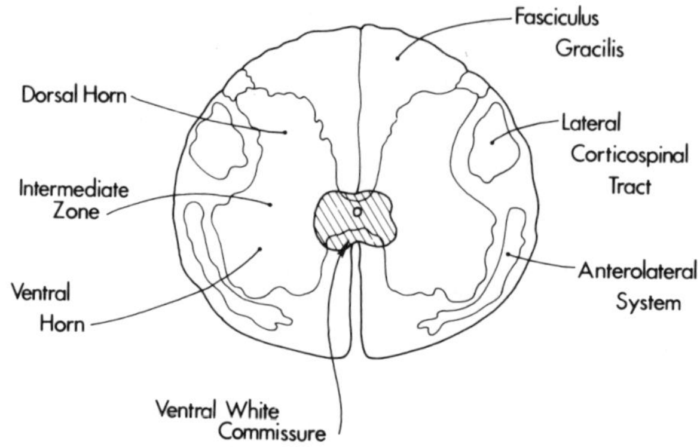

Fig. 1-17. SYRINGOMYELIA AT L_2 - L_5: A cavitation of the central areas of the cord at lumbar levels will cause characteristic deficits based on the structures and levels involved.

DEFICIT	ASSOCIATED STRUCTURE
A.	A. Ventral white commissure
B.	B. Lamina X of spinal grey

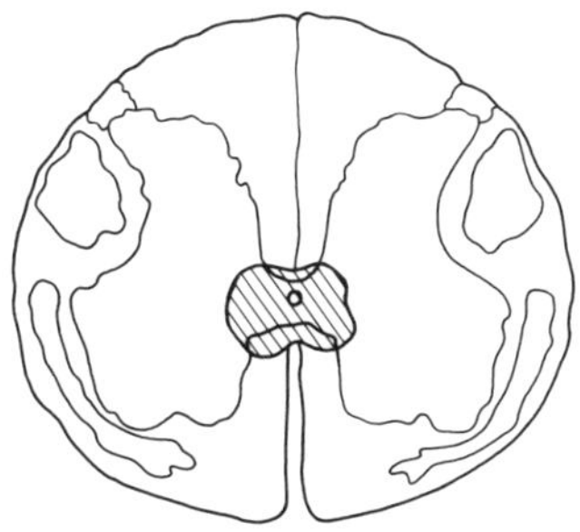

Fig. 1-18. Trajectory of fibers responsible for the symptoms seen in a syringomyelia at L_2 - L_5.

TRACT/FIBERS	RELATIONSHIP TO LESION	
	CELLS OF ORIGIN	TERMINATION

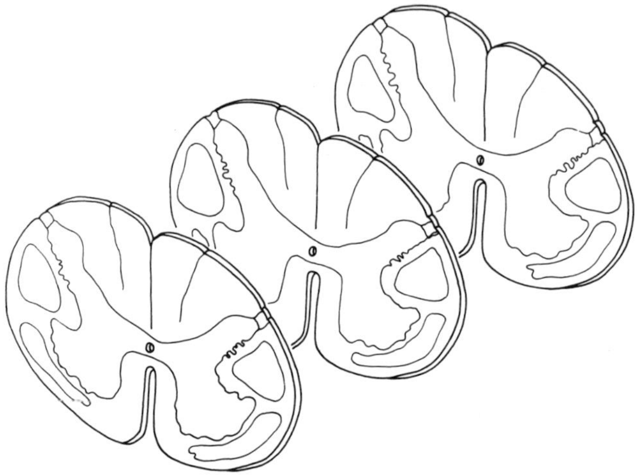

Fig. 1-19. Blank master drawing representative of cervical levels. This illustration can be used to outline lesions and correlate the subsequent deficits with specific structures.

DEFICIT

ASSOCIATED STRUCTURE

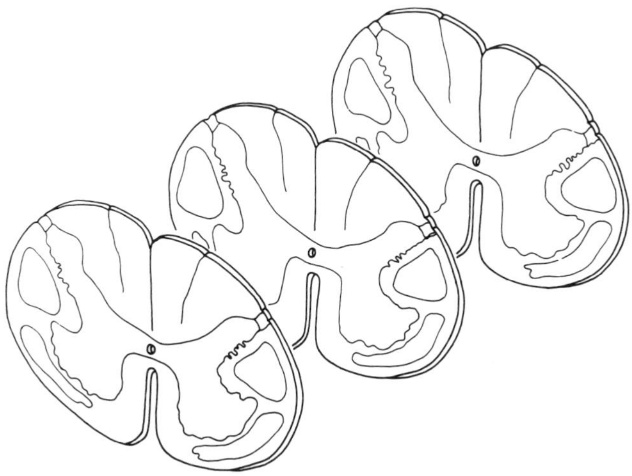

Fig. 1-20. This illustration is a companion to that shown in Fig. 1-19 and may be used to outline the trajectory of fibers through lesions outlined thereon.

	RELATIONSHIP TO LESION	
TRACT/FIBERS	CELLS OF ORIGIN	TERMINATION

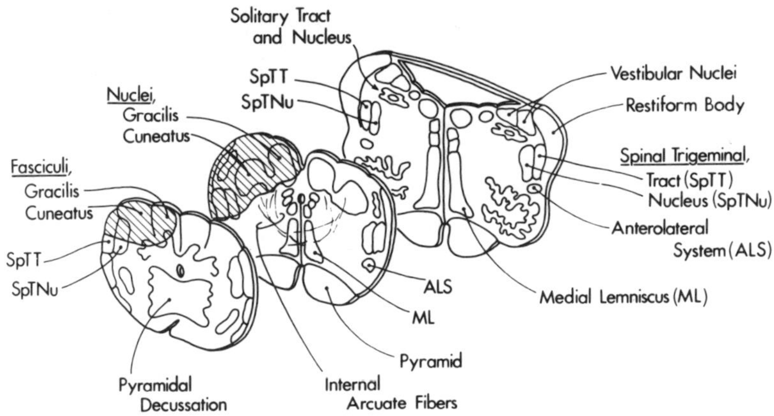

Fig. 2-1. LESION OF THE DORSOLATERAL MEDULLA: This could result from a traumatic insult or a vascular (posterior spinal artery) insufficiency.

DEFICIT	ASSOCIATED STRUCTURE
A. Ipsilateral loss of position and vibratory sense and touch over entire body below neck	A. Fasciculi and nuclei gracilis and cuneatus (dorsal column tracts and nuclei)
B. Ipsilateral loss of pain and temperature sensation over most of face, mouth, teeth and nasal cavity	B. Spinal trigeminal tract and nucleus

COMMENT: The partial sparing of ventral portions of the spinal trigeminal tract may result in some retention of sensation of the forehead. The face is represented in the spinal trigeminal tract and nucleus in an inverted pattern, the mandibular division representation is dorsal, the ophthalmic division is ventral and the maxillary division lies between these two.

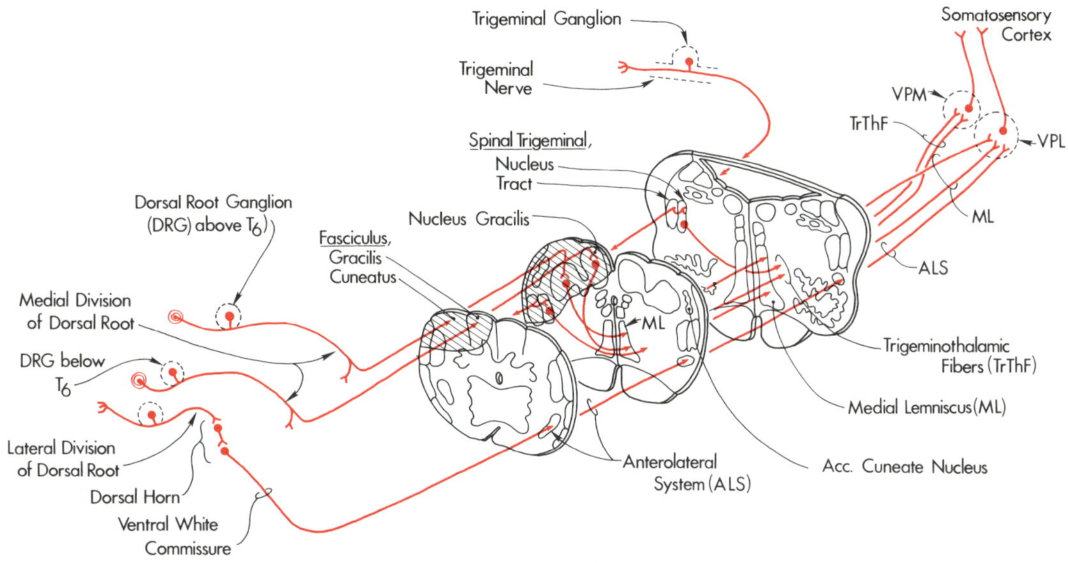

Fig. 2-2. Trajectory of fibers and locations of cells responsible for the symptoms seen in a lesion of the dorsolateral medulla.

	RELATIONSHIP TO LESION	
TRACT/FIBERS	CELLS OF ORIGIN	TERMINATION
A. Nuclei cuneatus and gracilis		
-Afferents	From ipsilateral dorsal root ganglia	Ipsilateral dorsal column nuclei (in lesion)
-Efferents	Cells in the dorsal column nuclei (in lesion)	Contralateral VPL of thalamus via medial lemniscus
B. Spinal trigeminal nucleus		
-Afferents	From ipsilateral trigeminal ganglion (also ganglia of cranial nerves VII, IX and X)	Ipsilateral spinal trigeminal nucleus (in lesion)
-Efferents	Cells in spinal trigeminal nucleus	Contralateral VPM of thalamus via ventral trigeminothalamic fibers

COMMENT: Although the lesion would involve dorsal spinocerebellar fibers and olivocerebellar fibers as they course through the restiform body, no obvious cerebellar deficit would result. Cuneocerebellar fibers (not shown) from the ipsilateral accessory cuneate nucleus to the ipsilateral anterior lobe cortex would also be injured as they course into the cerebellum. Note that the fibers of the anterolateral system are outside the area of the lesion. Consequently, pain and temperature input from the body, in contrast to the face, is intact.

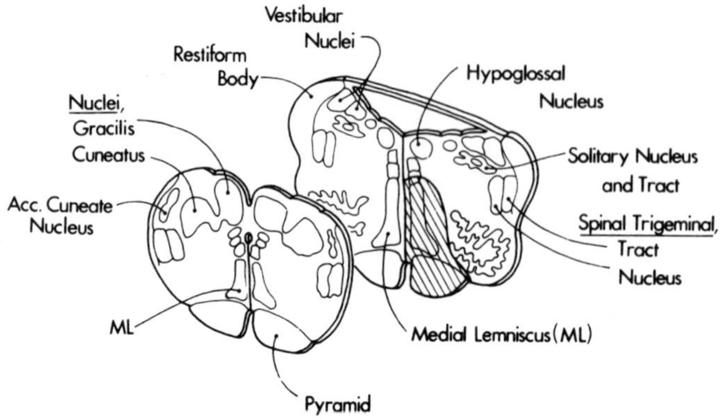

Fig. 2-3. MEDIAL MEDULLARY SYNDROME: This may result from an infarct due to a thrombosis of penetrating branches of the anterior spinal artery, the entire anterior spinal artery, or the vertebral artery. Occlusion of the vertebral artery may produce a wider range of symptoms including additional somatosensory (exteroceptive) losses.

DEFICIT	ASSOCIATED STRUCTURE
A. Contralateral loss of position and vibratory sense and discriminative touch over entire side of body	A. Medial lemniscus
B. Contralateral flaccid hemiplegia of upper and lower extremities, decreased reflexes, Babinski sign	B. Pyramid (corticospinal fibers)
C. Ipsilateral paresis (or paralysis) of tongue; on protrusion tongue will deviate toward side of lesion	C. Intramedullary hypoglossal rootlets

COMMENT: This lesion produces what is sometimes referred to as an inferior alternating hemiplegia due to the fact that one component of the paralysis is ipsilateral to the lesion (hypoglossal loss) while the other motor deficit is seen on the contralateral side (corticospinal loss). Since penetrating branches of the anterior spinal artery frequently serve the hypoglossal nucleus, the paralysis of the tongue may be a reflection of damage to the nucleus as well as to the rootlets; the effects are the same. Chronic lesions in this area may, with time, show a spastic paralysis of the extremities, weakness and hyperreflexia. This is presumably due to a spread of the lesion and subsequent involvement of descending extrapyramidal fibers.

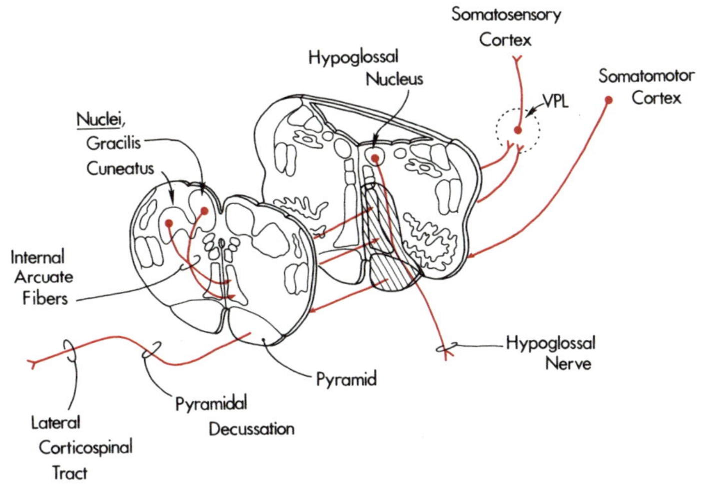

Fig. 2-4. Trajectory of fibers responsible for the symptoms seen in a medial medullary syndrome.

TRACT/FIBERS	RELATIONSHIP TO LESION	
	CELLS OF ORIGIN	TERMINATION
A. Medial lemniscus	Contralateral nuclei gracilis and cuneatus	Ipsilateral VPL of thalamus
B. Corticospinal fibers in pyramid	Ipsilateral somatomotor cortex	Contralateral spinal gray matter
C. Hypoglossal rootlets	Ipsilateral hypoglossal nucleus	Ipsilateral muscles of tongue (intrinsic, plus styloglossus, genioglossus and hyoglossus)

COMMENT: In some instances the lesion may cross the midline to involve portions of the contralateral medial lemniscus and/or pyramid. In such cases the loss may be more pronounced on one side and less on the other side.

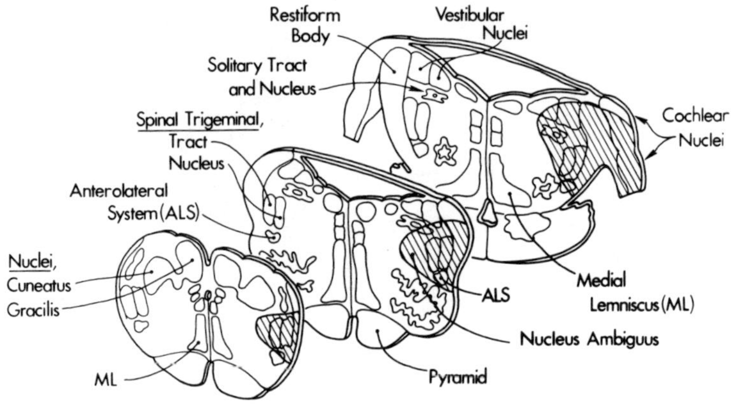

Fig. 2-5. LATERAL MEDULLARY SYNDROME (ALSO CALLED WALLENBERG'S SYNDROME): This is usually seen as a result of an infarct due to thrombosis of posterior inferior cerebellar or vertebral arteries. All or some of the deficits seen in this syndrome may be transient or permanent depending on the severity and rapidity of the vascular insult.

DEFICIT	ASSOCIATED STRUCTURE
A. Contralateral loss of pain and temperature sensation on the body	A. Anterolateral system (spinothalamic fibers)
B. Ipsilateral loss of pain and temperature sensation on the face	B. Spinal trigeminal tract and nucleus
C. Difficulty in swallowing and speech	C. Nucleus ambiguus
D. Ipsilateral diminution or loss of hearing	D. Cochlear nuclei and their connections
E. Nystagmus, nausea, ataxia toward the side of the lesion	E. Vestibular nuclei and their connections
F. Ipsilateral ptosis, miosis, enophthalamos (Horner's syndrome), diminution of sweating	F. Autonomic fibers descending through area of lesion

COMMENT: This is the most common of the medullary syndromes seen as a sequel to vascular lesions.

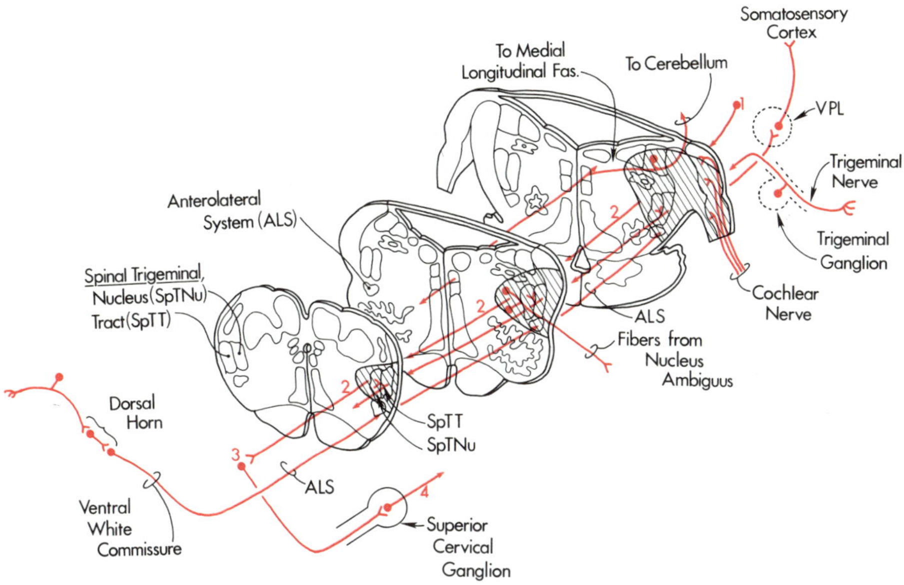

Fig. 2-6. Trajectory of fibers and location of cells responsible for the symptoms seen in an infarct due to thrombosis of the posterior inferior cerebellar artery (lateral medullary syndrome).

	RELATIONSHIP TO LESION	
TRACT/FIBERS	CELLS OF ORIGIN	TERMINATION
A. Anterolateral system	Contralateral laminae I-VI of spinal gray	Ipsilateral VPL of thalamus
B. Spinal trigeminal tract	Ipsilateral trigeminal ganglion (also ganglia of VII, IX and X - not shown)	Ipsilateral spinal trigeminal nucleus
C. Nucleus ambiguus in lesion	Nucleus ambiguus in lesion	Muscles of larynx and pharynx
D. Cochlear nuclei	Spiral ganglion (afferents), cochlear nuclei in lesion	Bilateral cochlear projections to auditory relay nuclei (not shown)
E. Vestibular nuclei	Vestibular ganglion (afferents), vestibular nuclei in lesion	Bilateral cerebellar cortex, motor nuclei of III, IV, VI, reticular formation

COMMENT: Horner's syndrome (ptosis, miosis, enophthalamos) is the result of the interruption of fibers which may originate from the reticular formation or hypothalamus (1), descend through the lesion (2), and terminate in the intermediolateral cell column (3). Preganglionic fibers enter the sympathetic chain, terminate in the superior cervical ganglion and postganglionic fibers (4) distribute to the head.

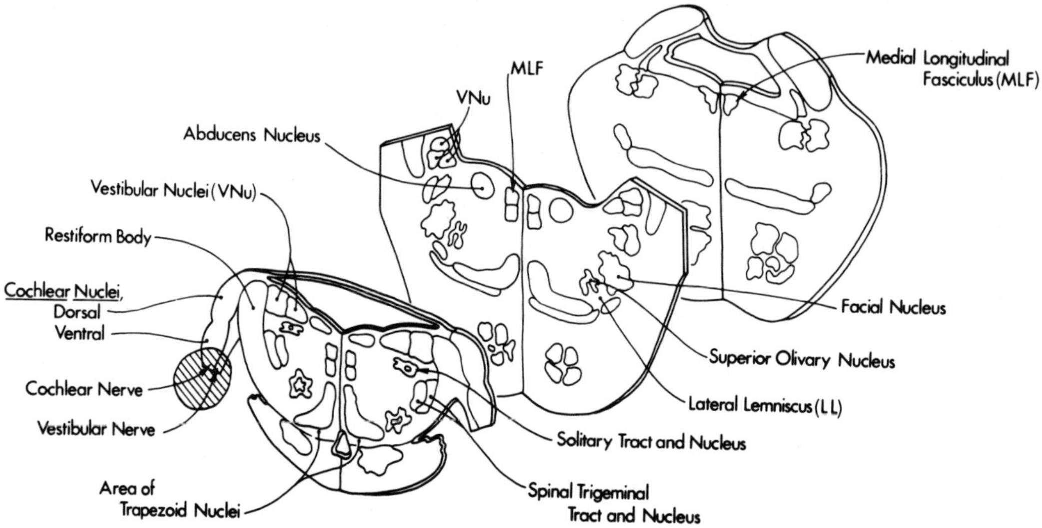

Fig. 2-7. EARLY (SMALL) ACOUSTIC NEUROMA: Acoustic neuromas presumably originate from Schwann cells located medial to the vestibular ganglion on the vestibular root of the eighth nerve. These tumors are most frequently found on the vestibular root within the internal auditory canal and meatus.

DEFICIT	ASSOCIATED STRUCTURE
A. Ipsilateral loss of hearing, tinnitus	A. Cochlear root of the eighth nerve
B. Unsteadiness, dizziness and possibly vertigo	B. Vestibular root of the eighth nerve

COMMENT: Although acoustic neuromas located within the internal auditory meatus may compress the facial and intermediate nerves, paresis of the facial muscles is rarely seen. Unusually observant individuals may notice a slight loss of taste sensations on the ipsilateral side of the tongue and less tearing in the ipsilateral eye.

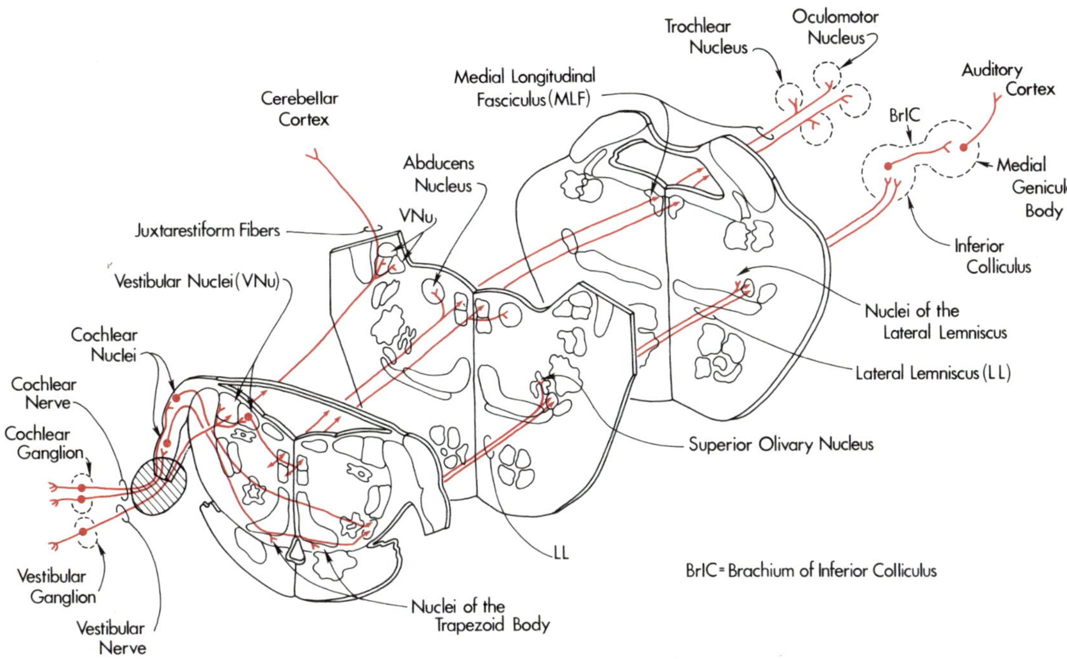

Fig. 2-8. Trajectory of fibers responsible for the symptoms seen in an early acoustic neuroma.

	RELATIONSHIP TO LESION	
TRACT/FIBERS	CELLS OF ORIGIN	TERMINATION
A. Cochlear root fibers	Ipsilateral spiral (cochlear) ganglion cells	Ipsilateral dorsal and ventral cochlear nuclei
B. Vestibular root fibers	Ipsilateral vestibular ganglion cells	Ipsilateral vestibular nuclei and cortex of the flocculonodular lobe of the cerebellum

COMMENT: Primary vestibulocerebellar fibers may also send collaterals into the medial (fastigial) and lateral (dentate) cerebellar nuclei. The vestibular nuclei project to cerebellar structures (secondary vestibulocerebellar fibers) as well as to the abducens, trochlear and oculomotor nuclei; the latter fibers course through the medial longitudinal fasciculus. Auditory data is relayed to the inferior colliculus, medial geniculate nucleus and the transverse temporal gyrus via multisynaptic bilateral pathways. Only crossed auditory projections are shown here.

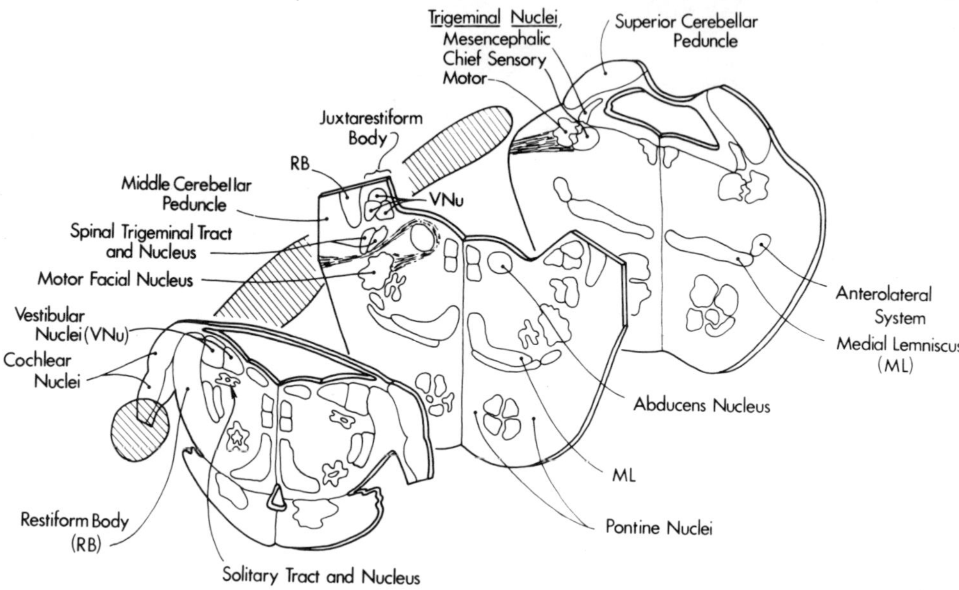

Fig. 2-9. LATE (LARGE) ACOUSTIC NEUROMA: Enlargement of an acoustic neuroma into the cerebellopontine angle may involve, in addition to the vestibular and cochlear roots (see Figs. 2-7, 2-8), the intracranial roots of the trigeminal and facial nerves, the cerebellar peduncles and portions of the cerebellar hemisphere is some cases.

DEFICIT	ASSOCIATED STRUCTURE
A. Ipsilateral loss, or depression, of corneal reflex, hypesthesia, paresthesia or loss of pain and temperature sensation on face	A. Trigeminal nerve at its exit from the pons
B. Ipsilateral loss of taste in anterior two-thirds of tongue, decrease in tearing, hypesthesia of external auditory canal	B. Facial nerve within the auditory canal and at its exit from the pons
C. Ipsilateral cerebellar signs; unstable gait, ataxia, dyssynergia, dysmetria, falling toward side of lesion	C. Cerebellar peduncles, inferior portions of the cerebellar hemisphere

COMMENT: A large acoustic neuroma will produce the above deficits, in addition, the cochlear and vestibular problems outlined in Figs. 2-7 and 2-8. Although this tumor may involve the motor roots of the facial and trigeminal nerves, corresponding motor deficits are not frequently seen. Careful testing of the corneal reflex will differentiate involvement of the sensory fibers of the trigeminal nerve versus the motor fibers of the facial nerve. Nystagmus is rarely seen as a spontaneous sign, however, it may be elicited by gaze in the horizontal plane.

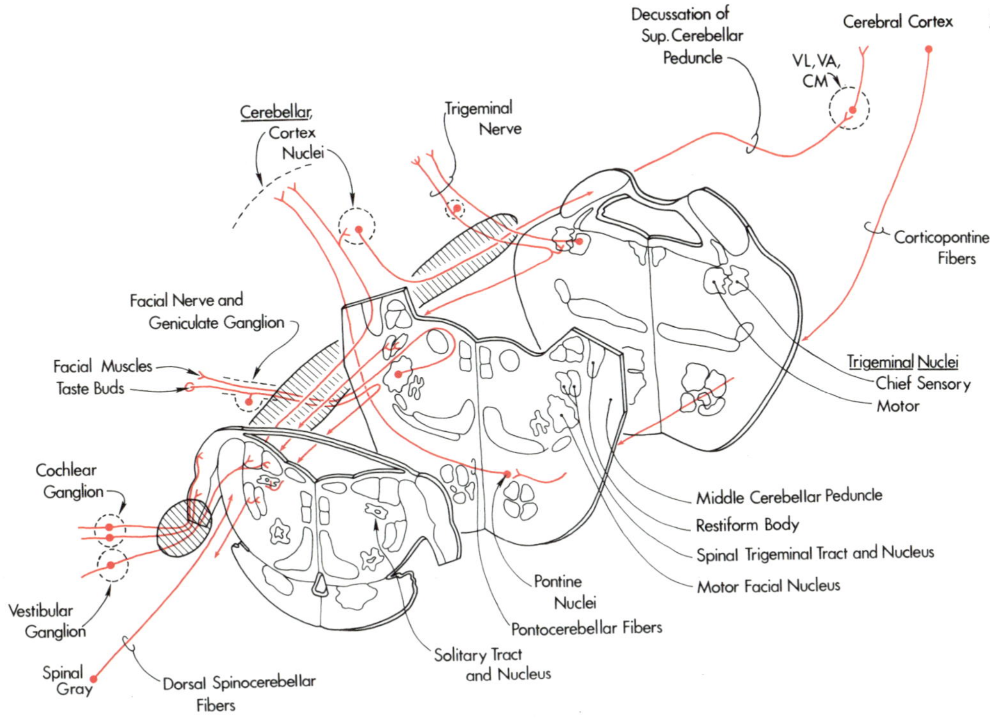

Fig. 2-10. Trajectory of fibers responsible for the symptoms seen in a late acoustic neuroma.

TRACT/FIBERS	RELATIONSHIP TO LESION: CELLS OF ORIGIN	TERMINATION
A. Trigeminal nerve, sensory root	Ipsilateral trigeminal ganglion	Ipsilateral chief sensory and spinal trigeminal nuclei
B. Facial nerve, intermediate part	Ipsilateral geniculate (facial) ganglion	Ipsilateral spinal trigeminal nucleus and solitary nucleus
	Ipsilateral superior salivatory nucleus	Ipsilateral pterygopalatine ganglion
C. Cerebellar peduncles		
-Restiform Body	Ipsilateral spinal cord	Ipsilateral cerebellum
	Contralateral olive	Ipsilateral cerebellum
-Middle	Contralateral pontine nuclei	Ipsilateral cerebellum
-Superior	Ipsilateral cerebellar nuclei	Contralateral thalamic nuclei

COMMENT: Only representative fibers coursing through the cerebellar peduncles are shown (see Figs. 5-1 to 5-6 for additional data). The cerebellum receives input from ipsilateral and contralateral centers and, by way of the projections of its nuclei, sends information to the contralateral motor cortex after relays in thalamic nuclei. The somatomotor cortex projects to the contralateral spinal cord. Lesions of the cerebellar peduncles and/or nuclei result in ipsilateral deficits (see also Chapter 5).

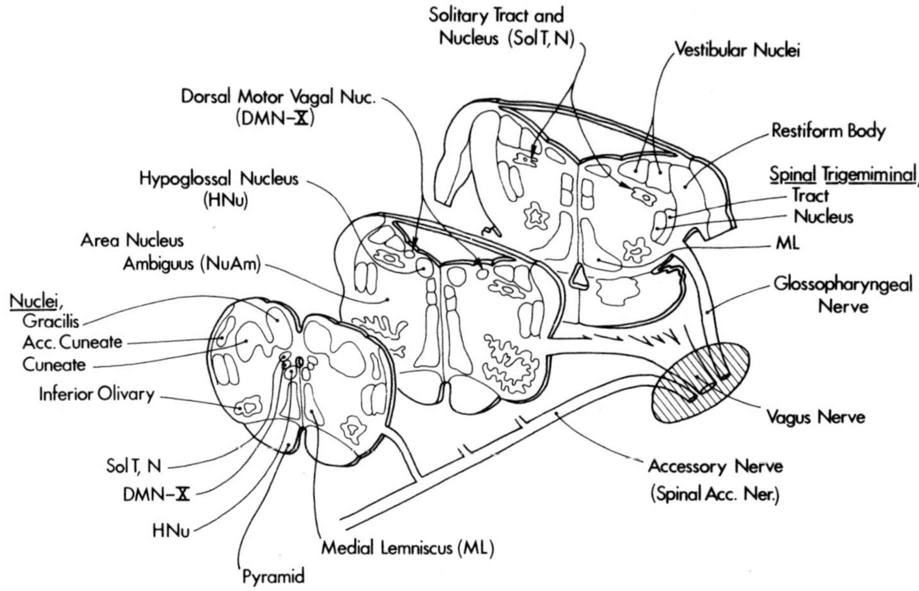

Fig. 2-11. LESION OF THE ROOTS OF THE GLOSSOPHARYNGEAL, VAGUS, AND SPINAL ACCESSORY NERVES (JUGULAR FORAMEN SYNDROME): Since these three cranial nerves exit through the jugular foramen they may be collectively involved in a tumor in this area, affected by disease processes such as subacute basilar meningitis, or involved in trauma.

DEFICIT	ASSOCIATED STRUCTURE
A.	A. Glossopharyngeal nerve.
B.	B. Vagus nerve.
C.	C. Spinal accessory nerve.

COMMENT: Tumors or other diseases of this general area of the posterior fossa may also involve the root of the hypoglossal nerve. Consequently, a lesion of the root of this nerve could be added to the above list.

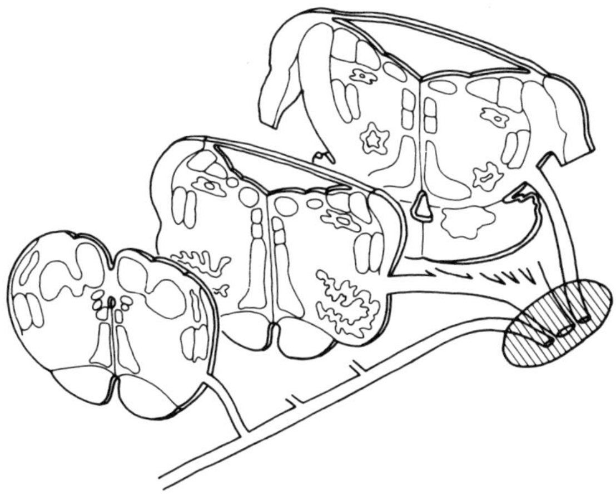

Fig. 2-12. Trajectory of fibers responsible for the symptoms seen in a lesion of the roots of the glossopharyngeal, vagus and spinal accessory nerves at the level of the jugular foramen.

TRACT/FIBERS	RELATIONSHIP TO LESION	
	CELLS OF ORIGIN	TERMINATION
A.		
B.		
C.		

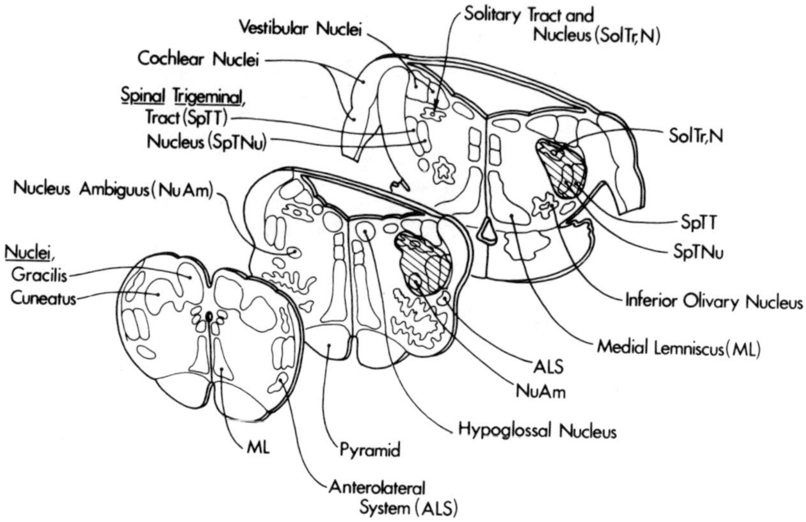

Fig. 2-13. LESION IN THE DORSOLATERAL AREA OF THE MEDULLA OBLONGATA: Small lesions in this general area are not common. The blood supply to this area is the posterior inferior cerebellar artery. This artery serves the solitary tract and nucleus and the spinal trigeminal tract and nucleus but not always the nucleus ambiguus. These structures collectively involved in a single lesion may be the result of a small glioma.

DEFICIT	ASSOCIATED STRUCTURE
A.	A. Solitary tract and nucleus
B.	B. Spinal trigeminal tract and nucleus
C.	C. Nucleus ambiguus

COMMENT: Note that the vestibular and cochlear nuclei are not involved and that the anterolateral system is intact. Compare the deficits seen in this example with those in Wallenberg's Syndrome.

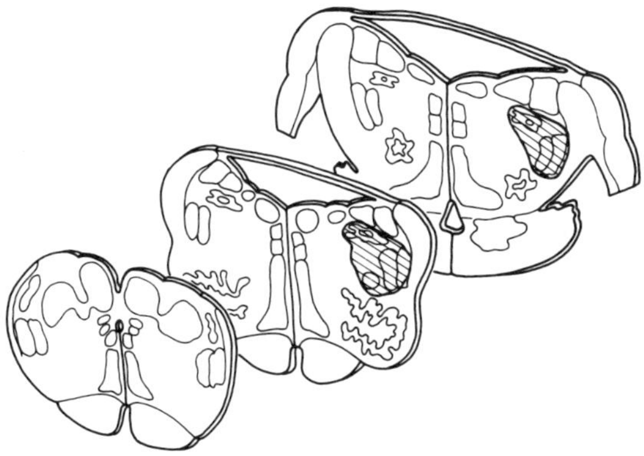

Fig. 2-14. Trajectory of fibers responsible for the symptoms seen in a lesion of the solitary tract and nucleus, the spinal trigeminal tract and nucleus, and the nucleus ambiguus.

TRACT/FIBERS	RELATIONSHIP TO LESION	
	CELLS OF ORIGIN	TERMINATION
A.		
B.		
C.		

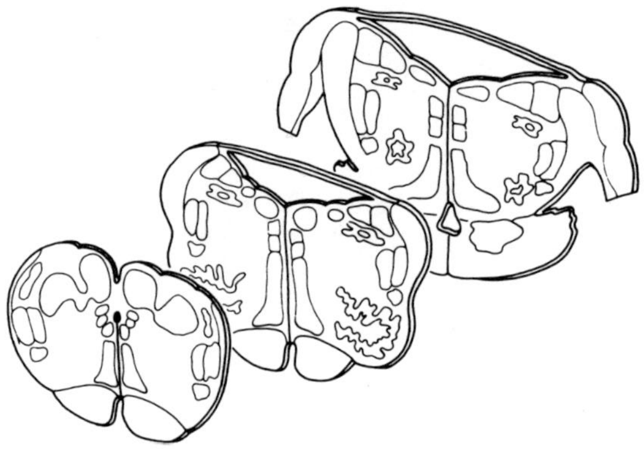

Fig. 2-15. Blank master drawing of representative levels through caudal, mid, and rostral medulla. This illustration can be used to outline lesions of the users choice and to correlate the appropriate deficits with specific structures.

DEFICIT	ASSOCIATED STRUCTURES

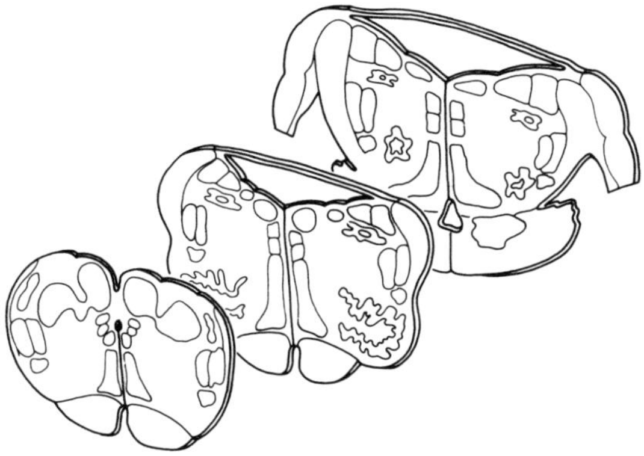

Fig. 2-16. This illustration is the companion to Fig. 2-15 and may be used to outline the trajectory of fibers through lesions outlined thereon.

TRACT/FIBERS	RELATIONSHIP TO LESION	
	CELLS OF ORIGIN	TERMINATION

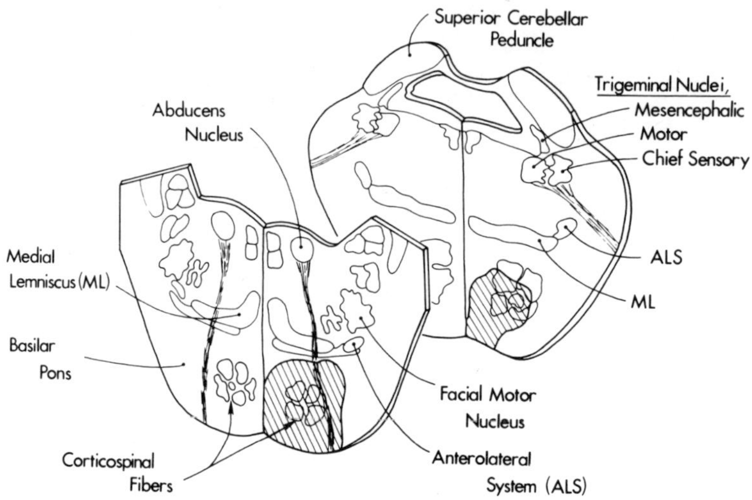

Fig. 3-1. MODIFIED MEDIAL PONTINE SYNDROME: May result from an infarct due to thrombosis of the paramedian branches of the basilar artery or from a tumor (e.g. glioma). This syndrome may also be seen subsequent to an aneurysm of the basilar artery at its junction with the vertebral. However, this may produce deficits which are, to varying degrees, bilateral.

DEFICIT	ASSOCIATED STRUCTURE
A. Ipsilateral flaccid paralysis of lateral rectus muscle; internal strabismus and inability to deviate eye laterally	A. Rootlets of abducens nerve in the basilar pons
B. Contralateral hemiplegia of upper and lower extremities, hyper-reflexia, hypertonia, Babinski sign	B. Corticospinal fibers in basilar pons

COMMENT: This particular deficit is sometimes referred to as a middle alternating hemiplegia for two reasons. First, it is midway (middle) between inferior (Fig. 2-3) and superior (Fig. 4-1) sites which also produce alternating motor losses. Second, one component of the paralysis is on the ipsilateral side (abducens loss) and the other component is on the contralateral side (corticospinal loss), hence the designation, alternating. Characteristic upper motor neuron signs are seen in chronic lesions. Initially there may be a flaccid hemiplegia, hypotonia and decreased reflexes.

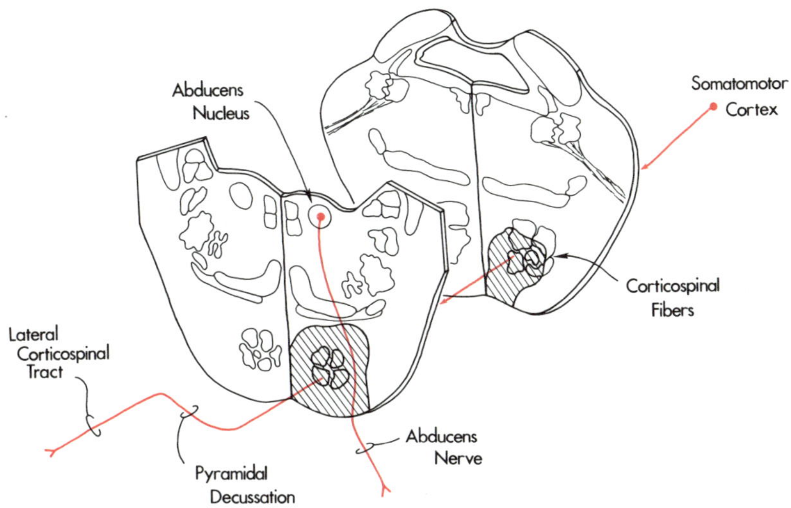

Fig. 3-2. Trajectory of fibers responsible for the symptoms seen in a medial pontine syndrome which involves only structures on one side of the midline.

	RELATIONSHIP TO LESION	
TRACT/FIBERS	CELLS OF ORIGIN	TERMINATION
A. Abducens rootlets	Ipsilateral abducens nucleus	Ipsilateral lateral rectus muscle
B. Corticospinal fibers	Ipsilateral somatomotor cortex	Contralateral spinal gray

COMMENT: These structures may also be involved in a tumor located in the basilar pons or may be damaged by pathologic alterations in the vascular system such as an aneurysm of the basilar artery. In the latter case deficits may be partially or symmetrically bilateral depending on the degree of insult. Proprioception, via the medial lemniscus, and exteroception, through the anterolateral system and trigeminothalamic fibers are intact. The spastic hemiplegia seen in chronic lesions is related to the involvement of descending extrapyramidal fibers.

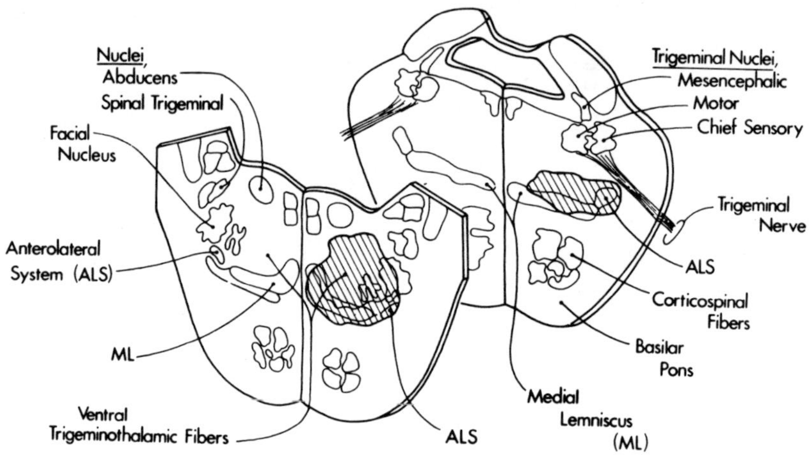

Fig. 3-3. GLIOMA OF THE PONTINE TEGMENTUM: Gliomas in the brainstem most frequently originate from anaplastic astrocytes, are usually highly invasive and can not be removed.

DEFICIT	ASSOCIATED STRUCTURE
A. Contralateral loss of position and vibratory sense and discriminative touch on arm, forearm and leg	A. Medial lemniscus
B. Contralateral loss of pain and temperature sensation on body	B. Anterolateral system (spinothalamic fibers)
C. Contralateral loss (or diminution) of pain and temperature sensation on face	C. Ventral trigeminothalamic fibers
D. Ipsilateral internal strabismus: paralysis of lateral rectus muscle	D. Rootlets from abducens nucleus in the pontine tegmentum
E. Ipsilateral flaccid paralysis, or paresis, of muscles of facial expression	E. Facial nucleus

COMMENT: Due to an interruption of descending input to medullary and spinal autonomic centers, components of a Horner's syndrome may also be present in a case with a glioma in the pontine tegmentum.

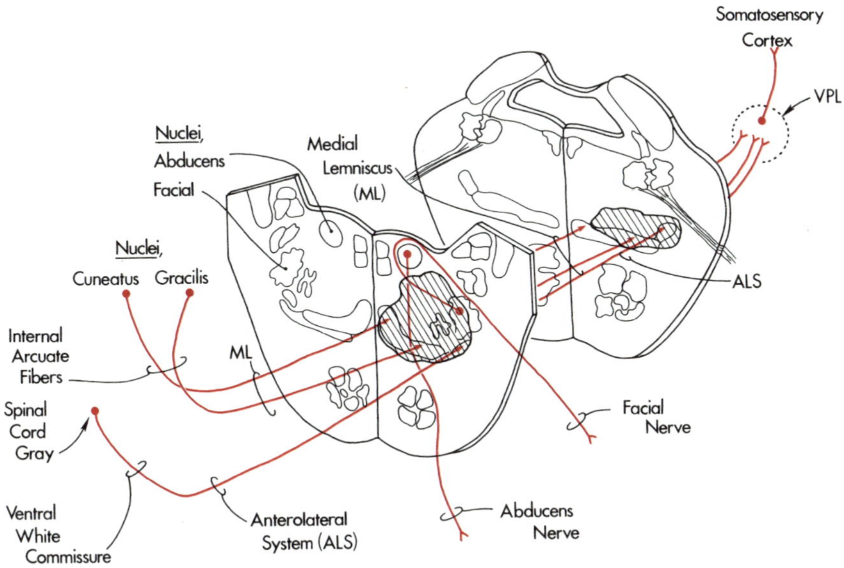

Fig. 3-4. Trajectory of fibers responsible for the symptoms seen in a glioma of the pontine tegmentum.

	RELATIONSHIP TO LESION	
TRACTS/FIBERS	CELLS OF ORIGIN	TERMINATION
A. Medial lemniscus	Contralateral nuclei cuneatus and gracilis	Ipsilateral VPL of thalamus
B. Anterolateral system	Contralateral laminae I-VI of spinal gray	Ipsilateral VPL of thalamus
C. Ventral trigemino-thalamic fibers (not shown)	Contralateral spinal trigeminal nucleus	Ipsilateral VPM of thalamus
D. Abducens rootlets	Ipsilateral abducens nucleus	Ipsilateral lateral rectus muscle
E. Facial nucleus	Ipsilateral motor facial nucleus (in lesion)	Ipsilateral muscles of facial expression

COMMENT: The course of trigeminothalamic fibers is not shown (see Figs. 2-2;3-8; 4-4). Depending on the extent of the lesion there may also be decreased tearing in the ipsilateral eye (visceral fibers of facial nerve) and/or an ipsilateral loss of taste from the anterior two-thirds of the tongue (special visceral afferent fibers).

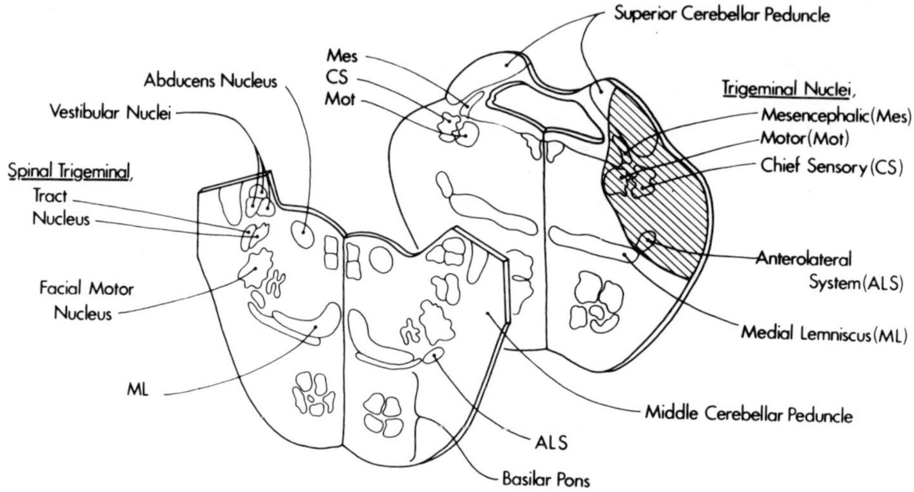

Fig. 3-5. **LESION OF THE DORSOLATERAL ASPECT OF THE ROSTRAL PONS:** This lesion is within the distribution areas of long circumferential branches of the basilar artery and branches of the superior cerebellar artery and may result from infarcts due to thromboses of these vessels. Gliomas or expanding tumors within the posterior fossa may also compromise this area.

DEFICIT	ASSOCIATED STRUCTURE
A. Contralateral loss of pain and temperature sensation on body	A. Anterolateral system (spinothalamic fibers)
B. Ipsilateral loss of pain, temperature sensation on face, and in oral and nasal cavities and loss of touch on face	B. Trigeminal root fibers, chief sensory nucleus, rostral parts of spinal trigeminal tract
C. Ipsilateral paralysis of muscles of mastication, jaw deviates toward side of lesion, atrophy of temporalis and masseter muscles	C. Motor trigeminal nucleus
D. Ipsilateral cerebellar signs	D. Superior cerebellar peduncle

COMMENT: Injury to the trigeminal root as it courses through the pons would also interrupt the sensory limb of the corneal reflex even though the motor limb (facial nucleus and nerve) is intact. Cerebellar signs are ipsilateral to the lesion and include intention tremor, ataxia (unsteady toward side of lesion), dyssynergia, dysdiadochokinesia, myoclonus, decomposition of movement, hypotonia, hyporeflexia, and in some cases a mild generalized weakness.

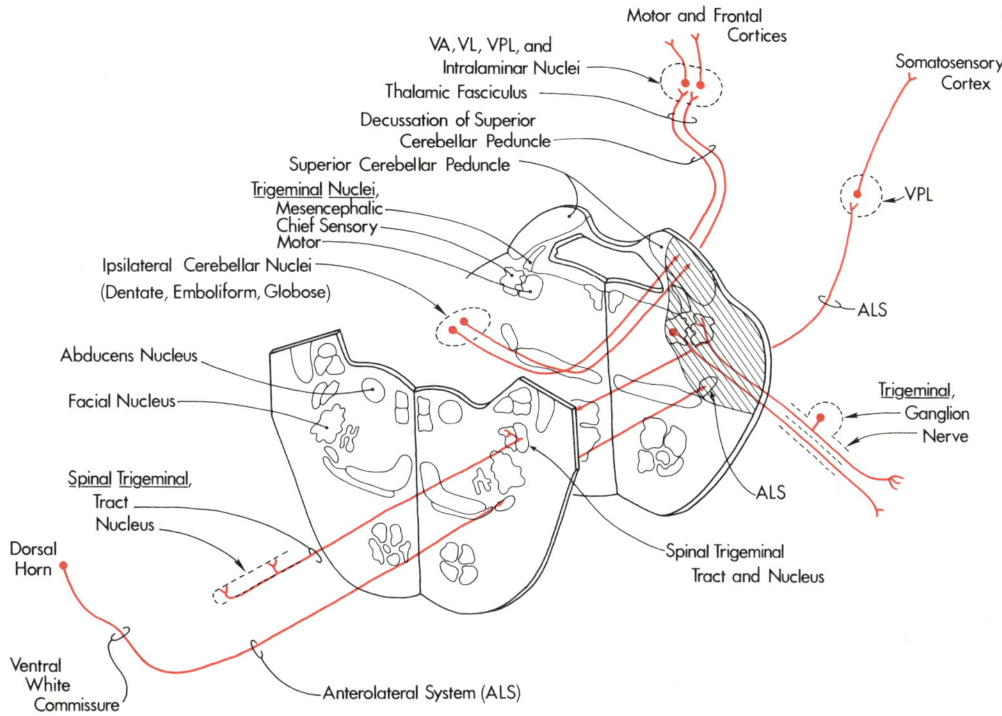

Fig. 3-6. Trajectory of fibers and locations of cells responsible for the symptoms seen in a lesion of the dorsolateral aspect of the pons at rostral levels.

	RELATIONSHIP TO LESION	
TRACT/FIBERS	CELLS OF ORIGIN	TERMINATION
A. Anterolateral system fibers	Contralateral spinal grav, laminae I-VI	Ipsilateral VPL of thalamus
B. Trigeminal root fibers, sensory portion	Ipsilateral trigeminal ganglion and mesencephalic nucleus	Ipsilateral chief sensory and spinal trigeminal nuclei
C. Trigeminal motor nucleus and efferent fibers	Ipsilateral trigeminal motor nucleus	Ipsilateral muscles of mastication, plus anterior belly of digastric, tensor tympani, tensor veli palatini, mylohyoid
D. Superior cerebellar peduncle	Ipsilateral dentate, globose, and emboliform cerebellar nuclei	Contralateral thalamic nuclei, red nucleus, reticular nuclei, inferior olivary complex (not all are shown)

COMMENT: Only representative targets of cerebellar nuclear efferents are listed. Although the lesion involves parts of the middle cerebellar peduncle, the cerebellar signs are related mainly to the injury to the superior peduncle.

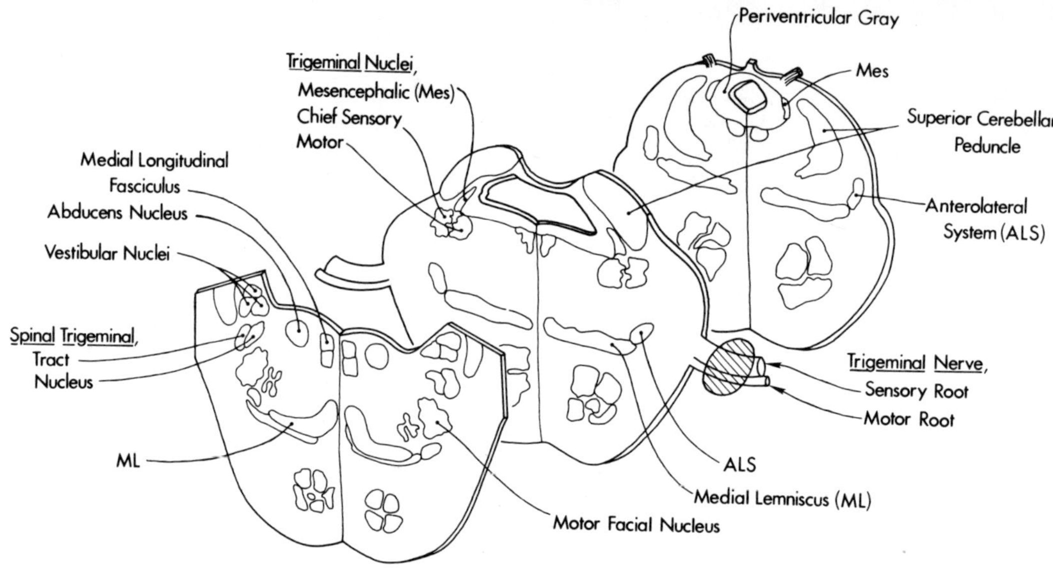

Fig. 3-7. LESION OF THE ROOT OF THE TRIGEMINAL NERVE: Injury to the root of the trigeminal nerve may be the result of, for example, trauma to the head, aneurysms, meningitis, or tumors which, as they enlarge, compress the nerve root. Tumors which compress the trigeminal root will affect sensory fibers first and motor fibers last.

DEFICIT	ASSOCIATED STRUCTURE
A. Ipsilateral loss of pain and temperature sensation on face, rostral portions of tongue, teeth and gingiva, loss of touch on face and afferent limbs of corneal reflex and jaw jerk reflex	A. Trigeminal nerve, sensory root
B. Ipsilateral paralysis of muscles of mastication, muscle atrophy, deviation of jaw toward side of lesion	B. Trigeminal nerve, motor root

COMMENT: Sneezing reflexes may also be lost in a trigeminal root lesion since peripheral sensory branches innervate the nasal mucosa.

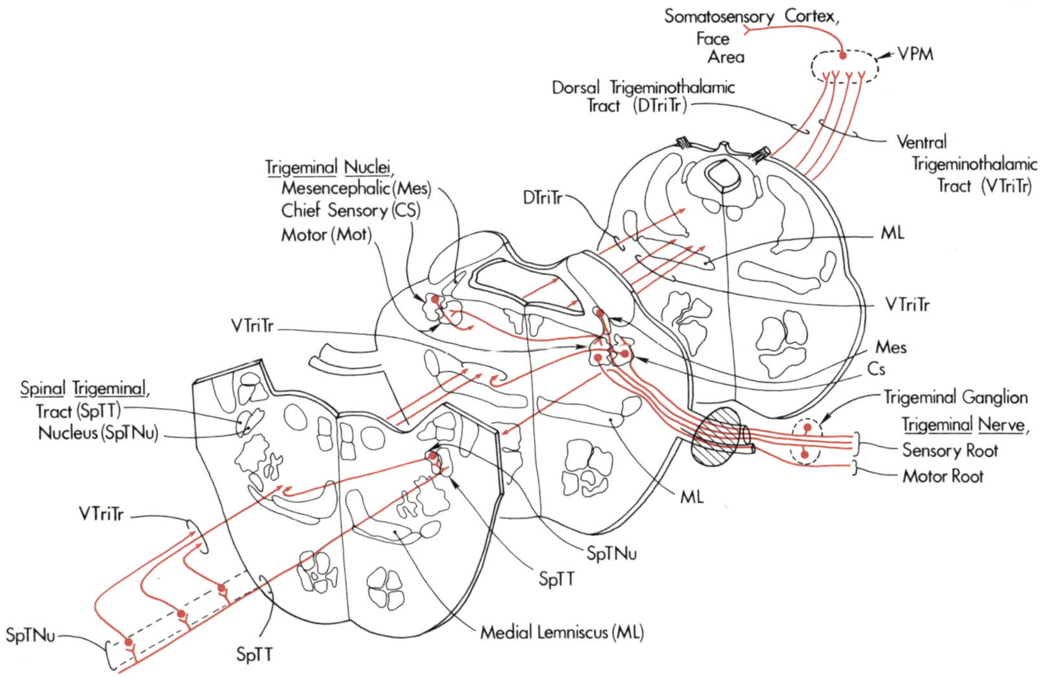

Fig. 3-8. Trajectory of fibers responsible for the symptoms seen in a lesion of motor and sensory roots of the trigeminal nerve.

	RELATIONSHIP TO LESION	
TRACT/FIBERS	CELLS OF ORIGIN	TERMINATION
A. Trigeminal nerve, sensory root	Ipsilateral trigeminal ganglion, cells of the mesencephalic nucleus	Ipsilateral chief sensory and spinal trigeminal nuclei, collateral fibers from mesencephalic nucleus to the trigeminal motor nuclei (jaw jerk reflex)
B. Trigeminal nerve, motor root	Ipsilateral trigeminal motor nucleus	Ipsilateral muscles of mastication, plus tensor tympani, tensor veli palatini, anterior belly of digastric, mylohyoid

COMMENT: Interruption of the afferent limb of the corneal reflex will be seen as analgesia of the cornea (no recognition of pain), however, the facial muscles (efferent limb) will function normally. On the drawing note, the trajectory of ventral trigeminothalamic fibers (crossed fibers arising in the spinal trigeminal and chief sensory nuclei) and dorsal trigeminothalamic fibers (uncrossed projections from the chief sensory nucleus).

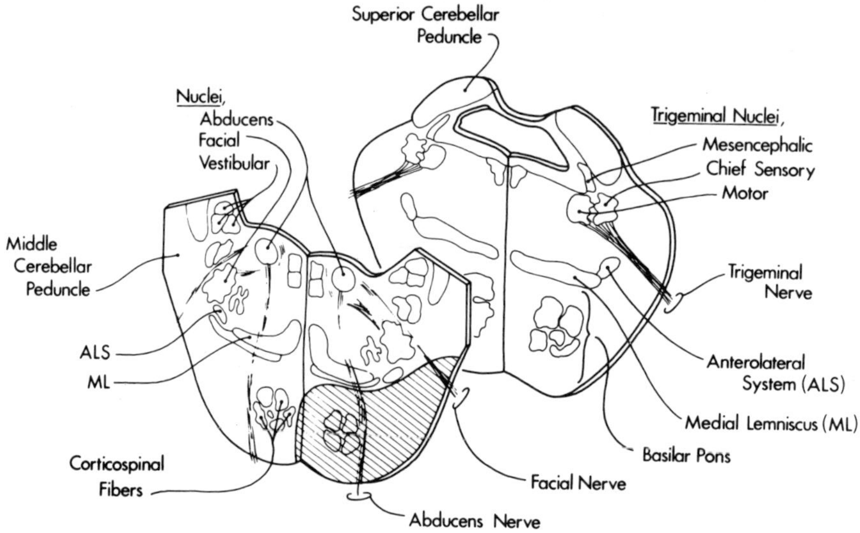

Fig. 3-9. MILLARD-GUBLER SYNDROME: This may result from an infarct due to thrombosis of paramedian and short circumferential branches of the basilar artery, from a large aneurysm of the basilar artery, or be seen in tumors originating within the basilar pons.

DEFICITS	ASSOCIATED STRUCTURE
A.	A. Corticospinal fibers
B.	B. Rootlets of the abducens nerve in the basilar pons
C.	C. Rootlets of the facial nerve in lateral aspects of the pons

COMMENT: Depending on the size of the lesion the medial lemniscus and larger parts of the middle cerebellar peduncle may also be involved. If this is the case there would be a contralateral loss of position and vibratory sense and touch (damage to medial lemniscus) and some ataxia ipsilateral to the lesion (damage to middle cerebellar peduncle). Such a lesion can be constructed on Figs. 3-15 and 3-16), or added to the above figure.

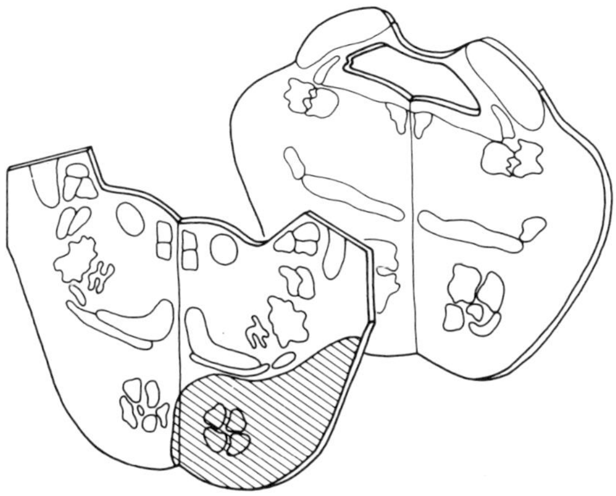

Fig. 3-10. Trajectory of fibers responsible for the symptoms seen in a Millard-Gubler syndrome as shown on the facing page.

TRACT/FIBERS	RELATIONSHIP TO LESION	
	CELLS OF ORIGIN	TERMINATION
A.		
B.		
C.		

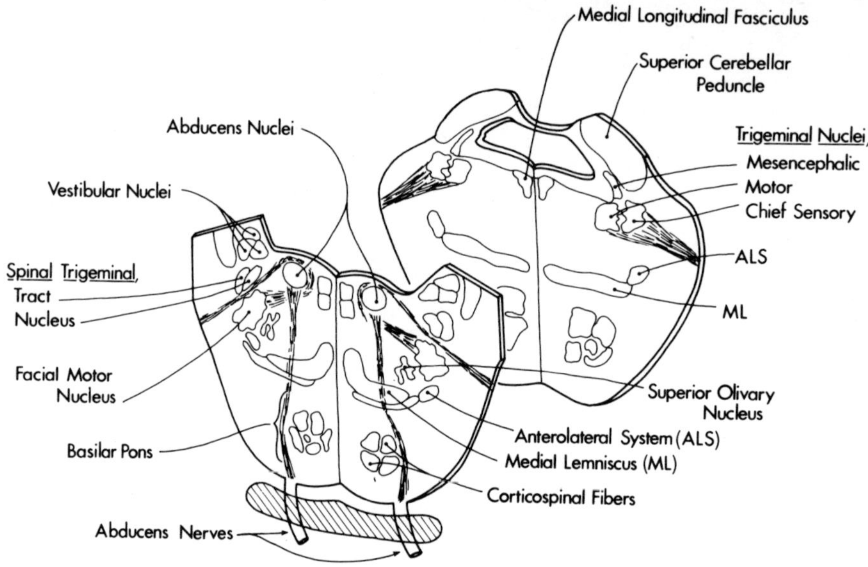

Fig. 3-11. BILATERAL DAMAGE TO THE ABDUCENS NERVES: Isolated lesions of the sixth cranial nerve may be seen in diabetes mellitus, chordoma, pontine glioma, trauma, and, when seen with other diagnostic signs, in cases where there is increased intracranial pressure. Such conditions may involve one or both nerves. The example shown here includes both nerves.

<u>DEFICIT</u>	<u>ASSOCIATED STRUCTURE</u>
A.	A. Roots of the abducens nerves

<u>COMMENT:</u> The long intracranial course of the abducens nerves makes them particularly susceptable to a variety of intracranial pathologic conditions.

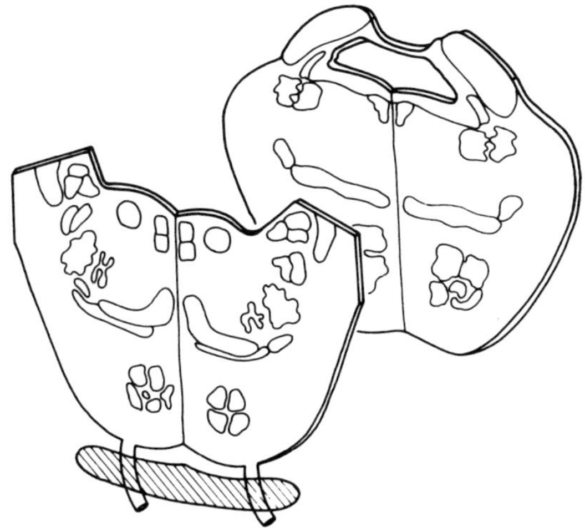

Fig. 3-12. Trajectory of fibers responsible for the symptoms seen in a bilateral lesion of the roots of the abducens nerves.

TRACT/FIBERS	RELATIONSHIP TO LESION	
	CELLS OF ORIGIN	TERMINATION
A.		

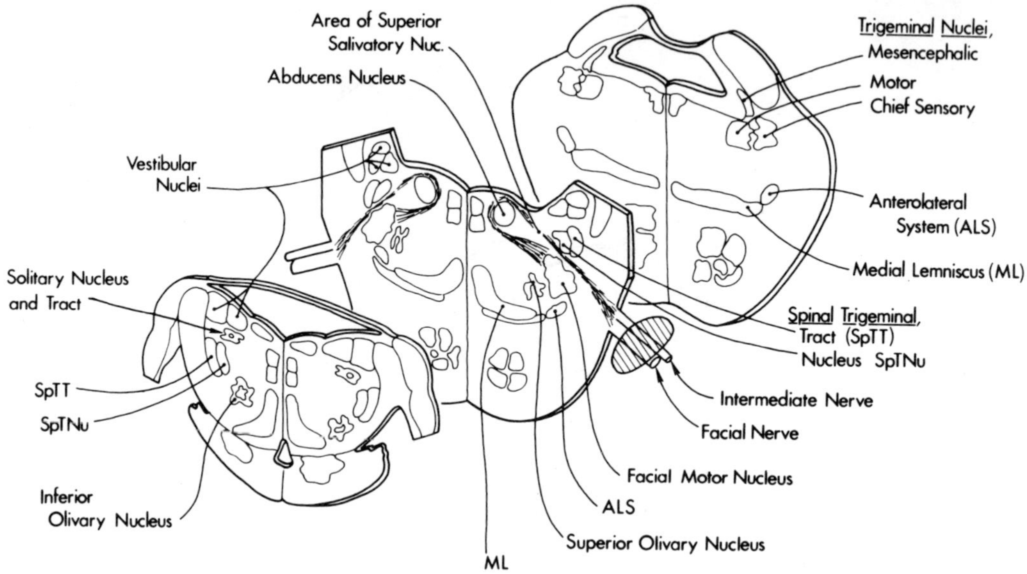

Fig. 3-13. LESION OF THE FACIAL NERVE: The seventh cranial nerve may be injured within the cranial cavity, along its course in the temporal bone, or at its exit from the stylomastoid foramen. Insults to the nerve may result from tumors, trauma to the face (lacerations of peripheral branches) or skull (fracture), aneurysms, meningitis, use of forceps during birth, or be seen as a sequel to a variety of other disease processes. Although the cause of Bell's palsy (idiopathic facial paralysis) is not known, it may be inflammatory in nature.

DEFICIT	ASSOCIATED STRUCTURE
A.	A. Facial nerve (motor and intermediate parts) at surface of brainstem

COMMENT: Compare the deficits that would be seen in, 1) a lesion of the facial nerve in the temporal bone proximal to the chorda tympani branch, and 2) a lesion of the facial nerve at the stylomastoid foramen with the deficits resulting in the example shown above. Damage at each of these sites will give specific signs and symptoms as correlated with the types of fibers damaged and the branching pattern of the nerve. Lesions of corticobulbar fibers en route to the facial motor nucleus will produce a paresis (or paralysis) of only the lower facial muscles contralateral to the lesion.

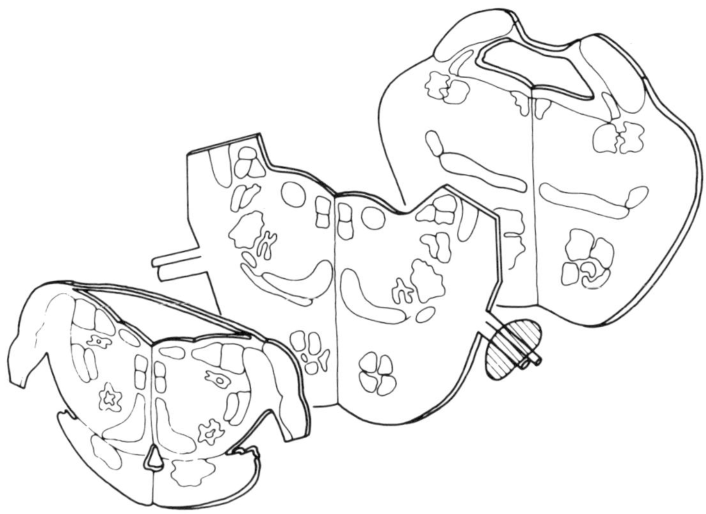

Fig. 3-14. Trajectory of fibers responsible for the symptoms seen in a lesion of the facial nerve (motor and intermediate parts).

TRACT/FIBERS	RELATIONSHIP TO LESION	
	CELLS OF ORIGIN	TERMINATION
A.		

COMMENT: The cells of the motor facial nucleus innervate facial muscles on the ipsilateral half of the face. Those parts of this nucleus which innervate muscles of the upper half of the face receive bilateral corticobulbar input while the portion of the nucleus that innervates muscles of the lower half of the face receives only contralateral input. These patterns explain the alternating losses when lesions interrupt corticobulbar fibers versus the motor root of the facial nerve.

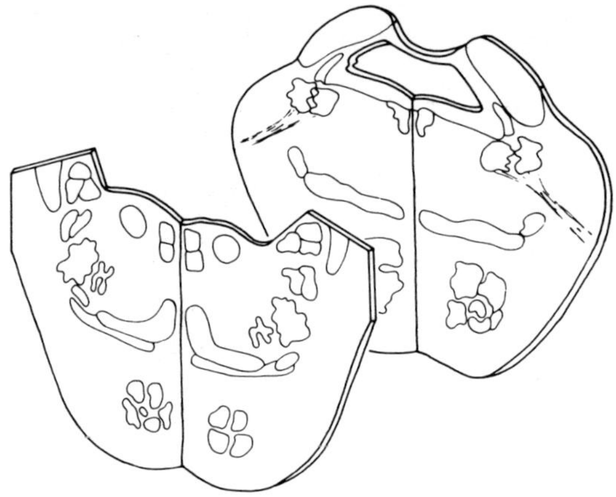

Fig. 3-15. Blank master drawing of representative levels through caudal (abducens, facial nuclei) and rostral (motor and chief sensory trigeminal nuclei) levels of pons. This illustration can be used to outline lesions of the user's choice and correlate the subsequent deficits with specific structures.

DEFICIT ASSOCIATED STRUCTURE

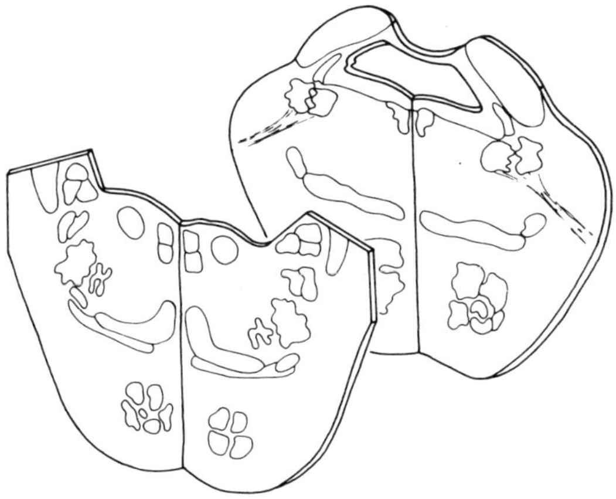

Fig. 3-16. This illustration is the companion to Fig. 3-15 and may be used to outline the trajectory of fibers passing though lesions outlined thereon.

	RELATIONSHIP TO LESION	
TRACT/FIBERS	CELLS OF ORIGIN	TERMINATION

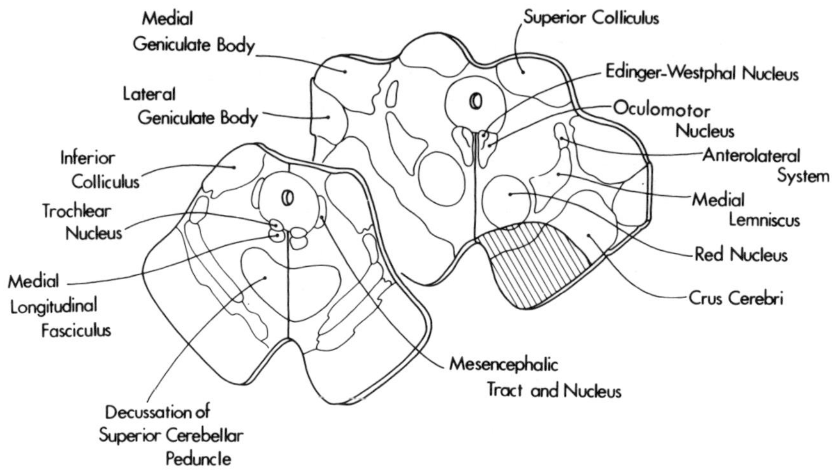

Fig. 4-1. WEBER'S SYNDROME: This may result from aneurysms of either the basilar bifurcation or proximal parts of the posterior cerebral artery. Similar deficits may also result from infarcts due to thrombosis of penetrating branches of the basilar bifurcation or the proximal segment of the posterior cerebral artery.

DEFICIT	ASSOCIATED STRUCTURE
A. Contralateral hemiplegia (or hemiparesis) of extremities, and Babinski sign	A. Corticospinal fibers in crus cerebri
B. Contralateral paresis (or paralysis) of muscles of facial expression on lower face, deviation of tongue to contralateral side	B. Corticobulbar fibers to motor facial nucleus and hyoglossal nucleus
C. Ipsilateral paralysis of most extraocular muscles, external strabismus and ptosis of eyelid, dilated pupil and absence of pupillary light reflex	C. Oculomotor rootlets

COMMENT: A Weber's syndrome that results from a vascular occlusion may be accompanied by contralateral cerebellar signs due to involvement of the red nucleus and adjacent ascending cerebellothalamic fibers. The lesion shown here produces a superior alternating hemiplegia. The oculomotor deficit is ipsilateral to the lesion while corticospinal and corticobulbar losses are seen on the contralateral side.

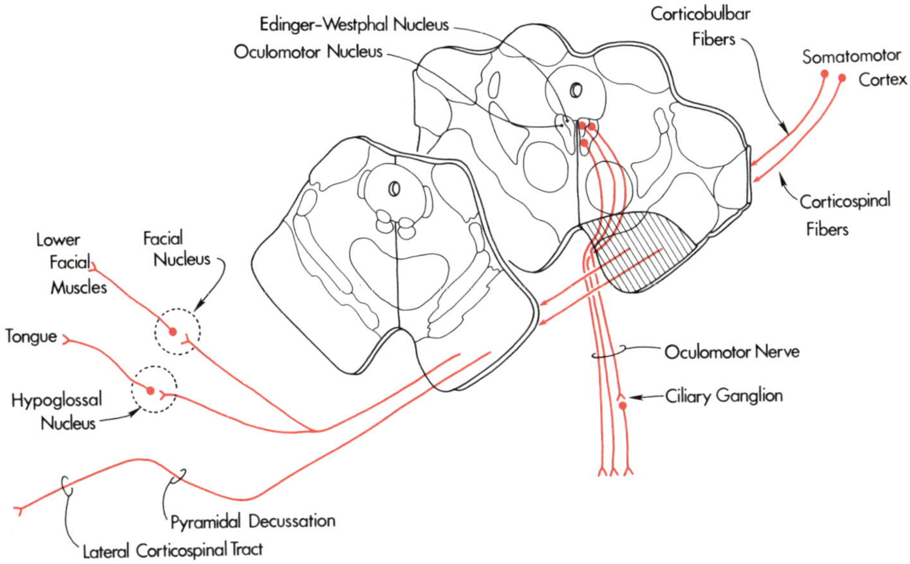

Fig. 4-2. Trajectory of fibers and locations of cells responsible for the symptoms seen in a lesion producing Weber's syndrome.

	RELATIONSHIP TO LESION	
TRACT/FIBERS	CELLS OF ORIGIN	TERMINATION
A. Corticospinal fibers	Ipsilateral somatomotor cortex	Contralateral spinal gray
B. Corticobulbar fibers	Ipsilateral somatomotor cortex	Contralateral parts of facial motor nucleus innervating lower half of face, parts of hypoglossal nucleus innervating genioglossus muscle
C. Oculomotor rootlets from:		
-Oculomotor nucleus	Ipsilateral oculomotor nucleus	Ipsilateral medial, superior and inferior recti muscles, inferior oblique and levator palpebrae muscles
-Edinger-Westphal nucleus	Ipsilateral E-W nucleus	Ipsilateral ciliary ganglion

COMMENT: Involvement of corticobulbar fibers in some cases may produce a deviation of the uvula toward the lesioned side on phonation.

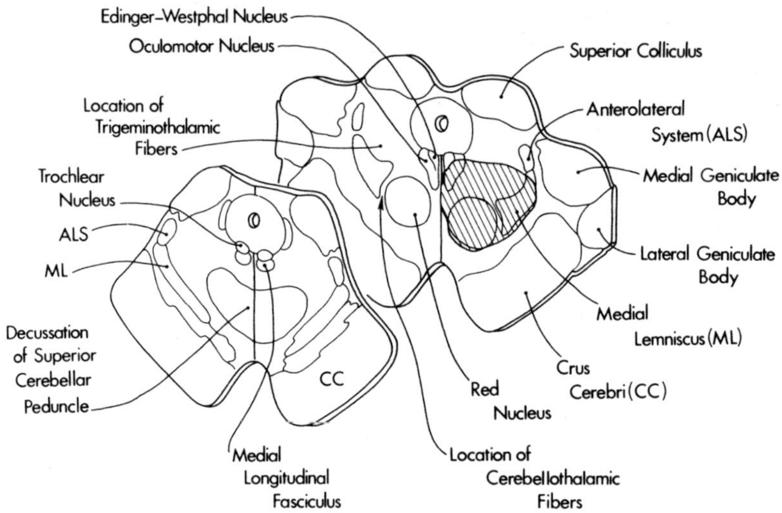

Fig. 4-3. GLIOMA OF THE MIDBRAIN TEGMENTUM: Gliomas most frequently originate from mature astrocytes. They are classified as grades I to IV based on their degree of anaplasia and mitotic activity (least to greatest).

DEFICIT	ASSOCIATED STRUCTURE
A. Contralateral loss of position and vibratory sense and discriminative touch	A. Medial lemniscus
B. Ipsilateral paresis (or paralysis) of most extraocular muscles, ptosis of eyelid, external strabismus, dilated pupil and loss of pupillary light reflex	B. Oculomotor rootlets coursing through the midbrain tegmentum
C. Contralateral loss of pain and temperature sensation from face	C. Ventral trigeminothalamic fibers
D. Contralateral cerebellar ataxia, intention tremor and other signs of the neocerebellar syndrome	D. Red nucleus, cerebellorubral fibers and cerebellothalamic fibers

COMMENT: A lesion which involves only the red nucleus, oculomotor rootlets and cerebellothalamic fibers is called Claude's syndrome.

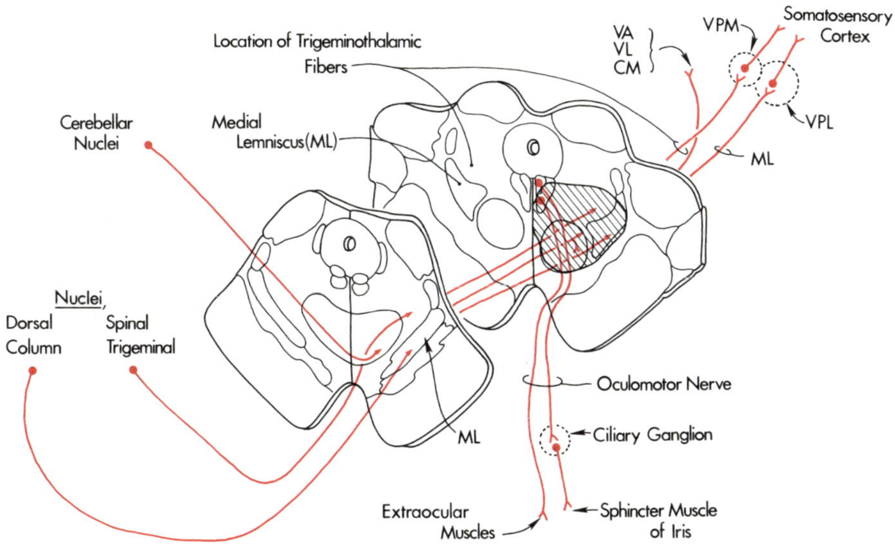

Fig. 4-4. Trajectory of fibers and locations of cells responsible for the symptoms seen in a glioma of the midbrain tegmentum.

	RELATIONSHIP TO LESION	
TRACT/FIBERS	CELLS OF ORIGIN	TERMINATION
A. Medial lemniscus	Contralateral nuclei gracilis and cuneatus	Ipsilateral VPL of thalamus
B. Oculomotor fibers from:		
-Oculomotor nucleus	Ipsilateral oculomotor nucleus	Ipsilateral superior, medial and inferior recti muscles, inferior oblique and levator palpebrae muscles
-Edinger-Westphal nucleus	Ipsilateral E-W nucleus	Ipsilateral ciliary ganglion
C. Ventral trigemino-thalamic fibers	Contralateral spinal trigeminal and chief sensory nuclei	Ipsilateral VPM of thalamus
D. Cerebellorubral and cerebellothalamic fibers	Contralateral dentate, emboliform and globose nuclei	Ipsilateral red nucleus and ventro-lateral, ventral anterior and centro-median nuclei of thalamus

COMMENT: Since there is sparing of the crus cerebri, no signs of corticospinal involvement are seen (compare with Weber's syndrome). Some fibers from the cerebellar nuclei also terminate in the oculomotor complex after crossing in the decussation of the superior cerebellar peduncle.

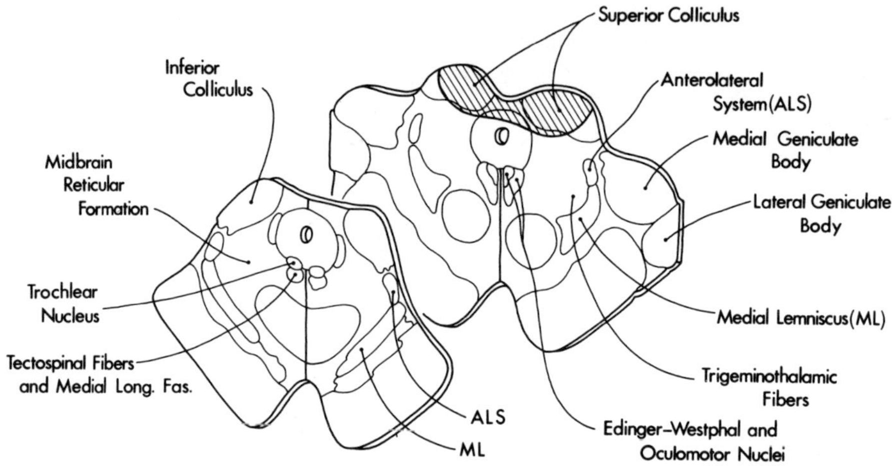

Fig. 4-5. PARINAUD'S SYNDROME (DORSAL MIDBRAIN SYNDROME): Tumors of the pineal (pinealoma) may be malignant or benign and are characterized by a wide variety of histologic features depending on their origin. Such tumors are a common cause of characteristic deficits in eye movement.

DEFICIT	ASSOCIATED STRUCTURE
A. Bilateral paresis of upward gaze above the horizontal plane, loss of convergence	A. Superior colliculus, compression or destruction

COMMENT: The example shown here illustrates involvement of the superior colliculi only. A pinealoma may also impinge on the pretectal area thus producing a bilateral loss (or irregularity) of the pupillary light reflex and accommodation. A diminution or loss of hearing may accompany involvement of the inferior colliculi. Enlargement of a pinealoma may compress the tectum and cause blockage of the cerebral aqueduct thereby producing signs of increased intracranial pressure (papilledema, headache, vomiting). Such signs are frequently seen in this syndrome.

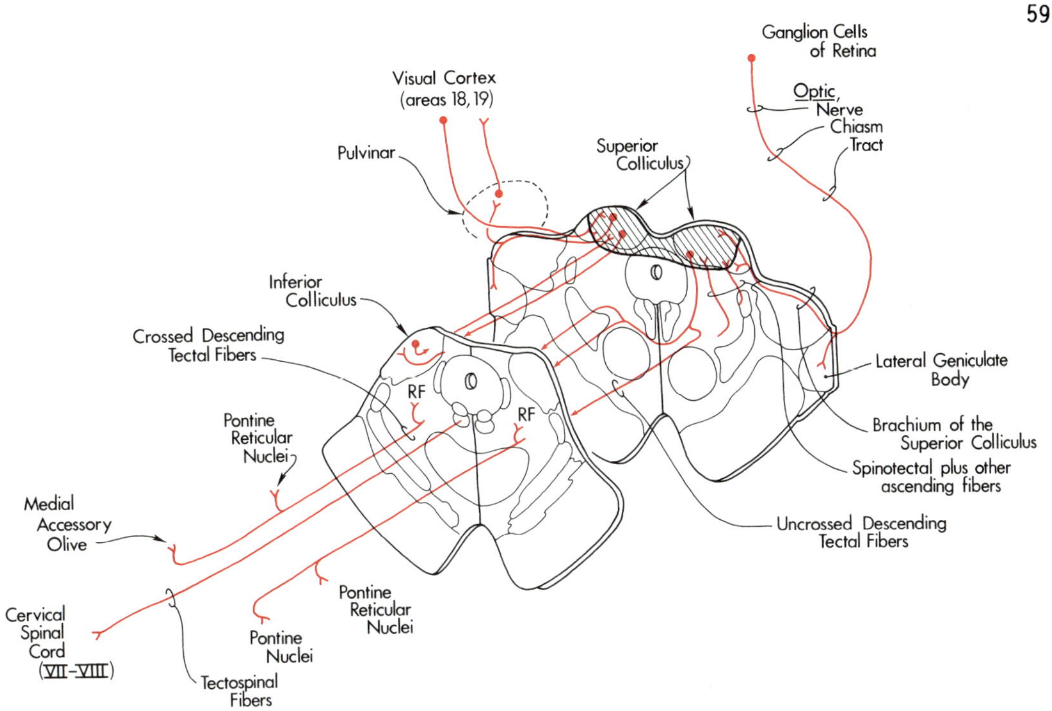

Fig. 4-6. Trajectory of fibers to and from the superior colliculus.

	RELATIONSHIP TO LESION	
TRACT/FIBERS	CELLS OF ORIGIN	TERMINATION
A. Superior colliculus, -Afferent fibers	Ganglion cells of retina	Superior colliculus, lateral geniculate body
	Inferior colliculus	Superior colliculus
	Areas 18, 19 of cerebral cortex	Superior colliculus
	Spinal cord via antero-lateral system (spino-tectal fibers)	Superior colliculus
B. Superior colliculus, -Efferent fibers	Superior colliculus	Pulvinar and lateral geniculate body
	Superior colliculus	Inferior colliculus
	Superior colliculus	Spinal cord (via tec-tospinal fibers) also reticular formation (midbrain and pons), pontine nuclei, and medial accessory olive

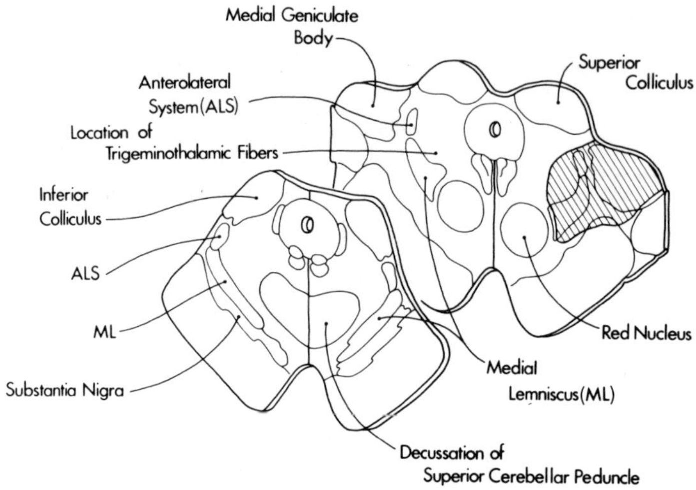

Fig. 4-7. LESION OF THE LATERAL MIDBRAIN TEGMENTUM AND ADJACENT MEDIAL GENICULATE NUCLEUS: This may result from a tumor in the region (e.g., glioma) or from an infarct due to thrombosis of some of the short circumferential branches of posterior cerebral or superior cerebellar arteries.

DEFICIT	ASSOCIATED STRUCTURE
A.	A. Anterolateral system
B.	B. Medial lemniscus
C.	C. Medial geniculate nucleus
D.	D. Some ventral trigeminothalamic fibers

COMMENT: Note the sparing of the crus cerebri, rootlets of the oculomotor nerve, cerebellorubral and cerebellothalamic fibers. The brachium of the superior colliculus overlies the medial geniculate and would be involved in the lesion.

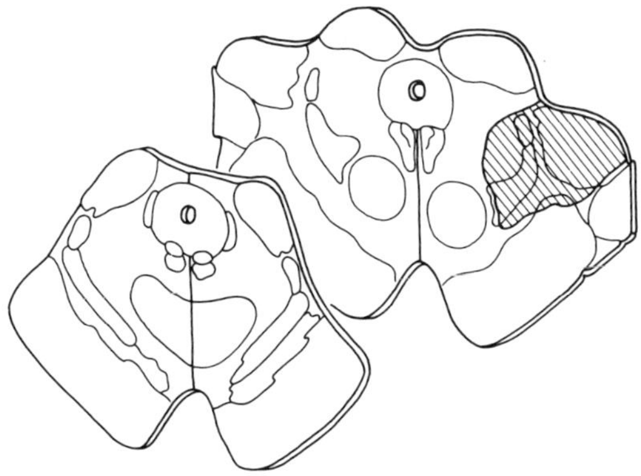

Fig. 4-8. Trajectory of fibers responsible for the symptoms seen in a lesion located in the lateral midbrain tegmentum and involving medial geniculate nucleus.

	RELATIONSHIP TO LESION	
TRACT/FIBERS	CELLS OF ORIGIN	TERMINATION
A.		
B.		
C.		
D.		

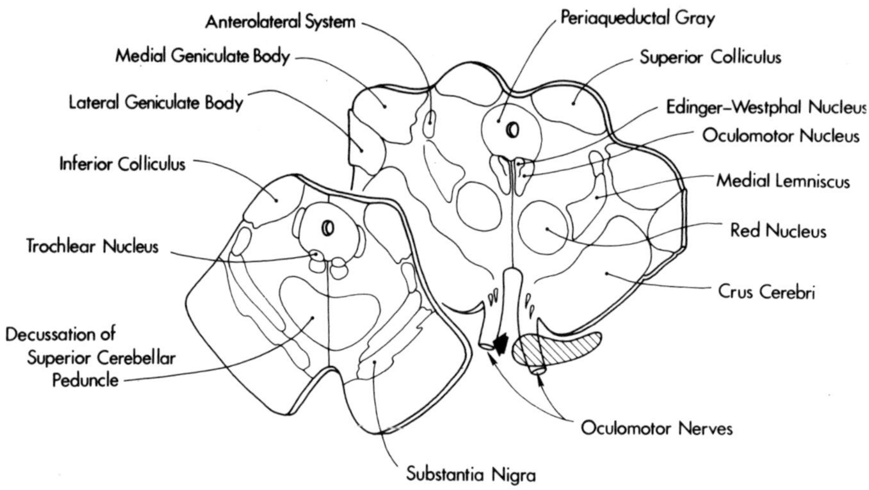

Fig. 4-9. LESION OF THE OCULOMOTOR NERVE: Injury to the third cranial nerve may be the result of aneurysms of the basilar bifurcation, hematomas (subdural or extradural), tumors along the route of the nerve, and basal meningitis. Ipsilateral or bilateral (large arrow) compression of the third nerve is frequently seen in medial herniation of the uncus consequent to an expanding supratentorial mass.

DEFICIT	ASSOCIATED STRUCTURE
A.	A. Oculomotor fibers to extraocular muscles
B.	B. Parasympathetic fibers from Edinger-Westphal nucleus to ciliary ganglion

COMMENT: Expanding tumors in supratentorial locations produce the cardinal signs of increased intracranial pressure (papilledema, headache, vomiting). Herniation of the uncus, seen as a sequel to the development of a tentorial pressure cone, may involve the third nerve ipsilaterally or bilaterally. In addition, there may be concomitant damage to the crus cerebri and the corticospinal and corticobulbar fibers contained therein. Compare the differences betwen a unilateral versus bilateral lesion of the root of the third cranial nerve.

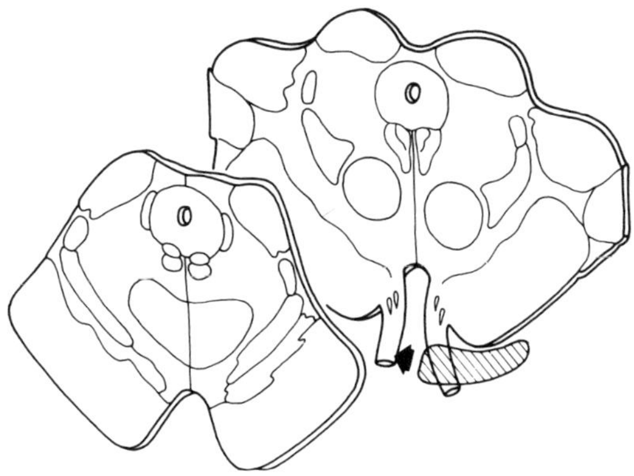

Fig. 4-10. Trajectory of fibers responsible for the symptoms seen in an ipsilateral or bilateral (large arrow) compression of the oculomotor nerve.

TRACT/FIBERS	RELATIONSHIP TO LESION: CELLS OF ORIGIN	RELATIONSHIP TO LESION: TERMINATION
A.		
B.		

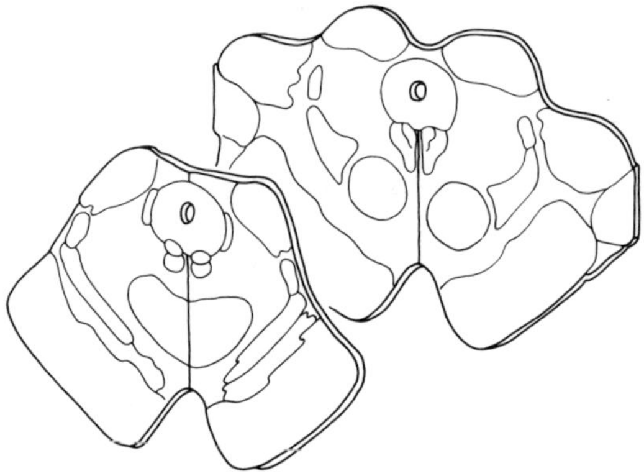

Fig. 4-11. Blank master drawing of representative levels through caudal (trochlear nucleus and decussation of the superior cerebellar peduncle) and rostral (oculomotor complex) levels of midbrain. This illustration can be used to outline lesions of the user's choice and to correlate the subsequent deficits with specific structures.

DEFICIT	ASSOCIATED STRUCTURE

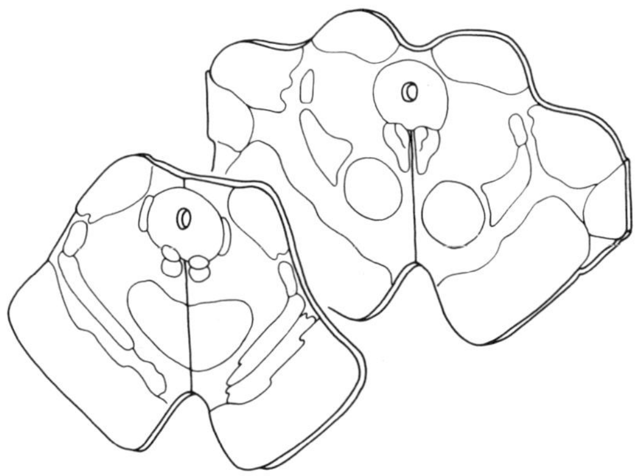

Fig. 4-12. This illustration is the companion to Fig. 4-11 and may be used to outline the trajectory of fibers passing through lesions outlined thereon.

TRACT/FIBERS	RELATIONSHIP TO LESION	
	CELLS OF ORIGIN	TERMINATION

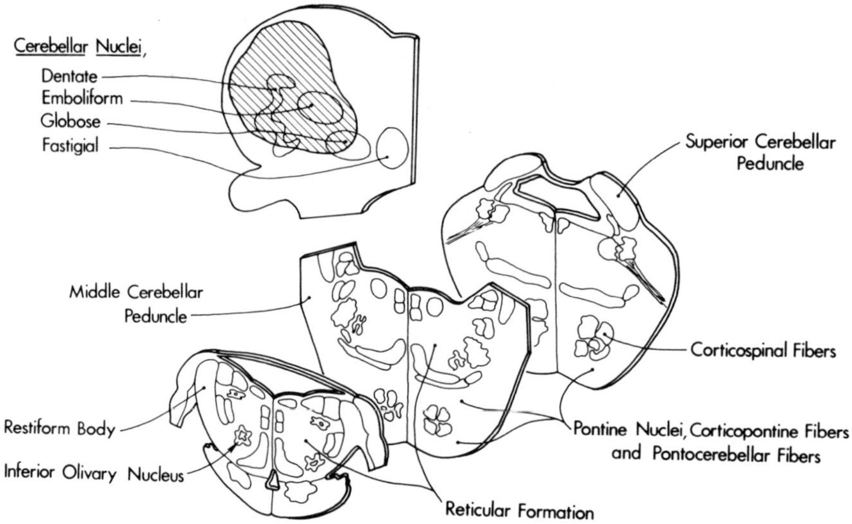

Fig. 5-1. LESION OF THE LATERAL (HEMISPHERE) PARTS OF THE CEREBELLUM: A lesion of lateral parts of the cerebellum will usually involve cortex as well as the dentate, emboliform and globose nuclei. Damage to this area of cerebellum may be the result of astrocytomas, trauma, hemangioblastomas, vascular disease and/or hemorrhage into the hemisphere, and infections (bacterial, viral, fungal) which may result in abscess formation.

DEFICIT	ASSOCIATED STRUCTURE
A. Ipsilateral hypotonia, intention tremor, dysmetria, dysdiadochokinesia, limb ataxia, rebound phenomenon, and some dysarthria	A. Lateral cerebellar cortex and dentate, emboliform and globose nuclei

COMMENT: Large lesions of only the cortex of the hemisphere do not cause significant deficits. Consequently, most types of cerebellar dysfunction are correlated with lesions of the nuclei or nuclei plus cortex. Mild gait ataxia and certain forms of nystagmus, although not common, may occasionally be seen in lesions of the cerebellar hemisphere. Large expanding tumors of the cerebellar hemisphere may also produce papilledema, a cardinal sign of increased intracranial pressure.

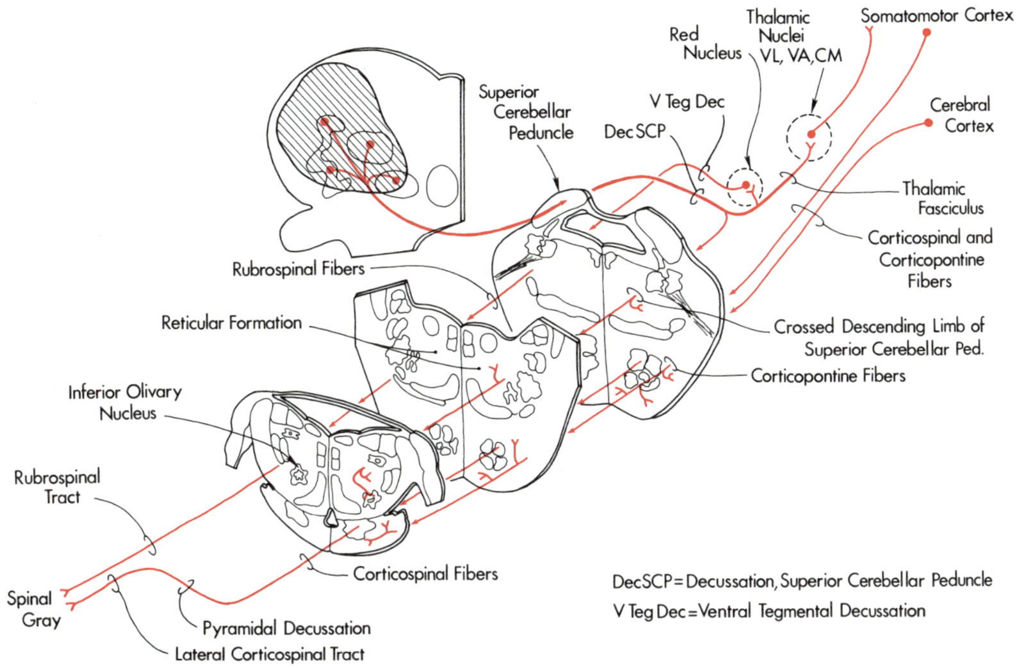

Fig. 5-2. Trajectory of fibers and locations of cells responsible for the symptoms seen in a lesion of lateral portions of the cerebellum (cortex plus dentate, emboliform, and globose nuclei). Since the deficits are related primarily to damage to the nuclei, only their basic efferent projections are shown (see Fig. 5-5 and 5-6 for selected afferents).

	RELATIONSHIP TO LESION	
TRACT/FIBERS	CELLS OF ORIGIN	TERMINATION
A. Cerebellar nuclear cells	Ipsilateral dentate, emboliform, globose nuclei	Contralateral red nucleus, VL, VA and CM thalamic nuclei, reticular formation, inferior olivary nuclei

COMMENT: Only representative targets of cerebellar efferent projections are shown; there are others. Note that information from the cerebellar nuclei is relayed mainly to the contralateral dorsal thalamus and from here on to the somatomotor cortex. Cells in the somatomotor cortex send their axons, as part of the corticospinal tract, through the brainstem and pyramidal decussation to the contralateral spinal cord. The decussation of cerebellar efferent fibers in the midbrain and the crossing of corticospinal fibers in the caudal medulla explains, in general terms, why the motor dysfunction seen following lesions of the cerebellar hemisphere are ipsilateral to the damaged area.

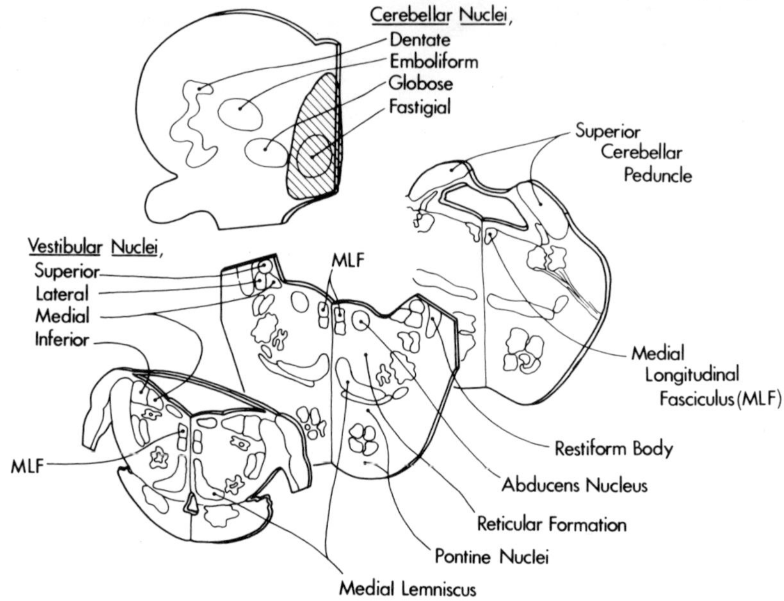

Fig. 5-3. LESIONS OF MIDLINE (VERMIS) PORTIONS OF THE CEREBELLUM: Lesions of midline regions of the cerebellum most frequently involve the fastigial nucleus and various portions of the vermal cortex of anterior and posterior lobes and the nodulus. Tumors which impinge on these structures are medulloblastomas (seen most frequent in children), ependymomas of the fourth ventricle, astrocytomas, and rarely papillomas of the choroid plexus.

DEFICIT	ASSOCIATED STRUCTURE
A. Truncal ataxia and instability, ataxia of gait, titubation, posturing of the head (head tilt), nystagmus, ocular dysmetria	A. Medial cerebellar cortex and fastigial nucleus

COMMENT: Mild dysarthria may also be seen following lesions of midline cerebellar structures. Limb ataxia, tremor, dysmetria and other signs of lateral cerebellar lesions are seldom seen in concert with the truncal ataxia and postural problems characteristic of midline cerebellar lesions. In addition, lesions of midline areas of cerebellum are usually bilateral.

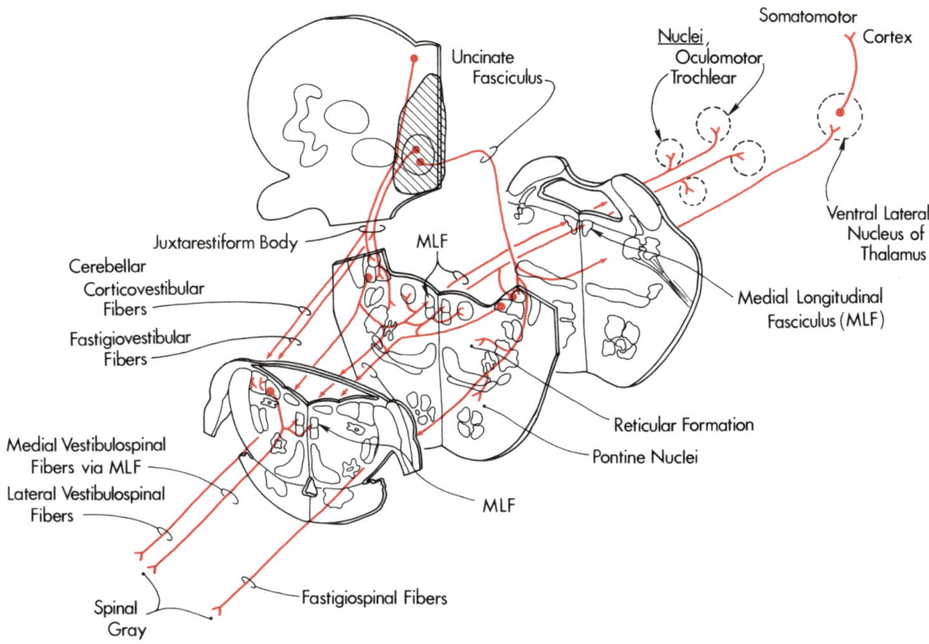

Fig. 5-4. Trajectory of fibers and location of cells responsible for the symptoms seen in a lesion of midline cerebellar structures (fastigial nucleus plus vermal cortex). Only efferent cortical and nuclear fibers are shown (see Fig. 5-5 and 5-6 for selected afferents).

	RELATIONSHIP TO LESION	
TRACT/FIBERS	CELLS OF ORIGIN	TERMINATION
A. Fibers from vermal cortex (cortico-vestibular fibers)	Ipsilateral Purkinje cells	Ipsilateral vestibular nuclei
B. Efferents of the fastigial nucleus	Ipsilateral fastigial nucleus in lesion	Ipsilateral vestibular nuclei; contralateral vestibular nuclei, reticular formation, spinal cord, and VL nucleus of thalamus

COMMENT: The vestibular nuclei receive bilateral input from the fastigial nucleus, project bilaterally to the cerebellar cortex and project to spinal centers via medial and lateral vestibulospinal tracts. The vestibular nuclei, subsequent to their receipt of bilateral fastigial input, also project bilaterally to the motor nuclei of the abducens, trochlear and oculomotor nerves via the medial longitudinal fasciculus. These general points (in addition to the bilateral nature of most lesions in this area), illustrate why there is bilateral truncal ataxia and pronounced nystagmus and other ocular deficits following damage to midline cerebellar structures. Cerebellar corticonuclear fibers, which project from the vermal cortex into the fastigial nucleus, are not shown.

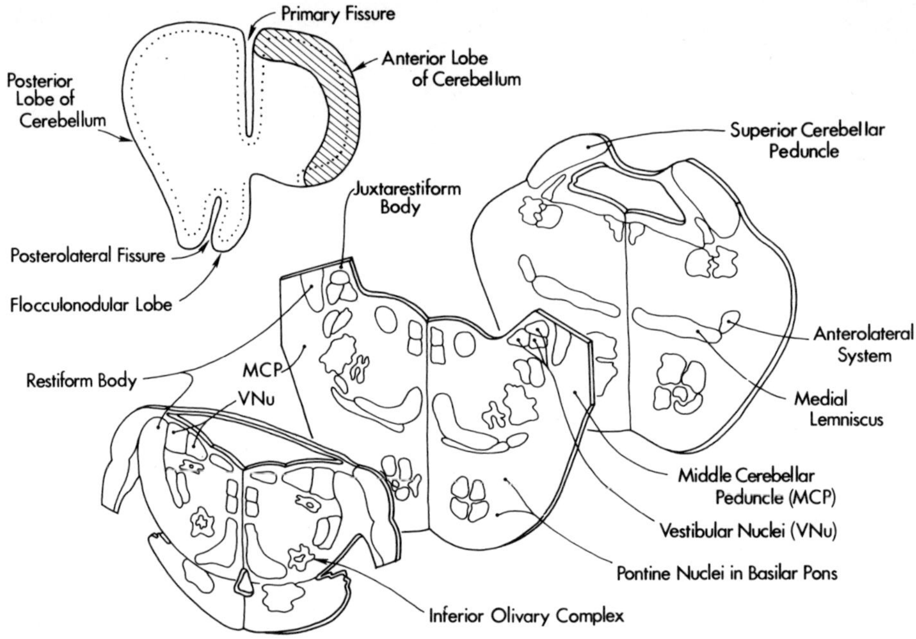

Fig. 5-5. ALCOHOLIC CEREBELLAR DEGENERATION: This disorder is most frequently seen in chronic alcoholics who have mild to severe malnutrition. The cerebellar deficits, once established, do not improve even with subsequent good nutrition and vitamin therapy.

DEFICIT	ASSOCIATED STRUCTURE
A. Severe gait ataxia (wide based, shuffling, unstable), titubation, truncal instability, incoordination of extremities (severe in lower, mild in upper)	A. Severe loss of neural cellular elements in the anterior lobe vermis, with milder loss in hemispheres

COMMENT: Neuronal loss involves all cellular elements of the anterior lobe with the Purkinje cells being the most severely affected. Although mild when compared to the cerebellar cortex, cell loss may also be seen in the emboliform, globose and fastigial nuclei, and in the inferior olivary complex and vestibular nuclei. Ocular motor problems, nystagmus and dysarthria are rarely seen. Slurred speech may be present but will usually disappear as the blood alcohol level decreases with time.

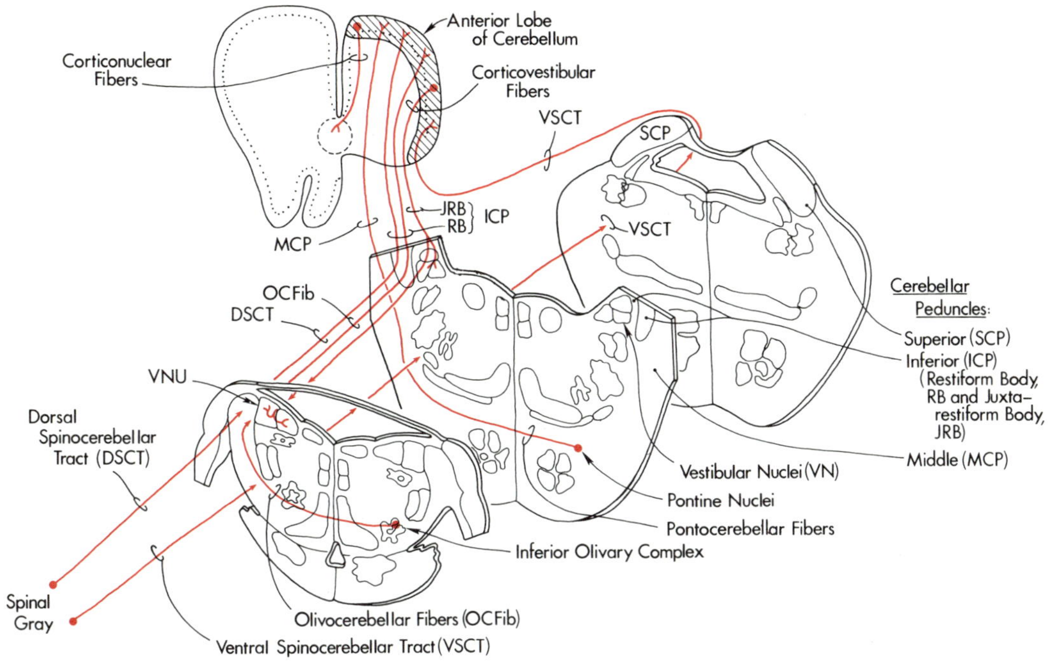

Fig. 5-6. Trajectory of fibers responsible for the symptoms seen in alcoholic cerebellar degeneration. Although there is cell loss in some precerebellar relay nuclei, the deficits are related primarily to cerebellar cortical degeneration. Selected afferent and efferent connections of the cortex are shown.

	RELATIONSHIP TO LESION	
TRACT/FIBERS	CELLS OF ORIGIN	TERMINATION
A. Dorsal spinocerebellar terminals	Ipsilateral dorsal nucleus of Clarke	Ipsilateral granular layer of cortex
B. Ventral spinocerebellar terminals	Bilateral spinal border cells and intermediate zone	Bilateral granular layer of cortex
C. Olivocerebellar terminals	Contralateral inferior olivary complex	Ipsilateral molecular layer of cortex
D. Pontocerebellar terminals	Contralateral pontine nuclei	Ipsilateral granular layer of cortex
E. Corticonuclear fibers	Ipsilateral Purkinje cells	Ipsilateral fastigial, emboliform, and globose nuclei
F. Corticovestibular fibers	Ipsilateral Purkinje cells	Ipsilateral vestibular nuclei

COMMENT: There is a minor ipsilateral pontocerebellar connection. Cell loss in the cerebellar nuclei, and in the inferior olivary complex and vestibular nuclei may be secondary to the destruction of their terminals in the anterior lobe cortex.

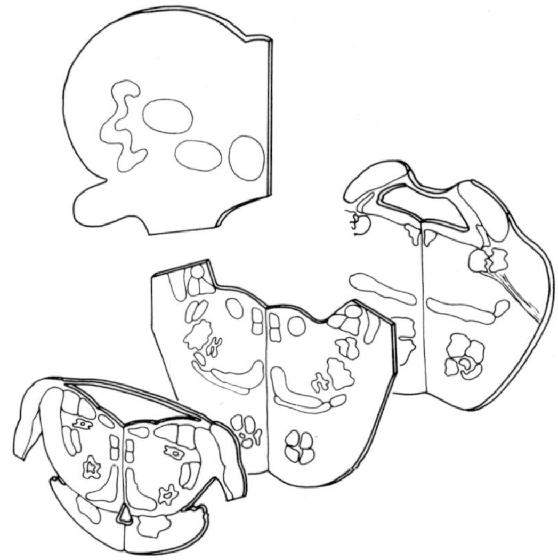

Fig. 5-7. Blank master drawing representative of the cerebellar cortex and nuclei and brainstem levels through the rostral medulla oblongata, caudal, and rostral pons. This illustration can be used to outline lesions of cerebellar structures and correlate the subsequent deficits with the involved structure.

<u>DEFICIT</u>	<u>ASSOCIATED STRUCTURE</u>

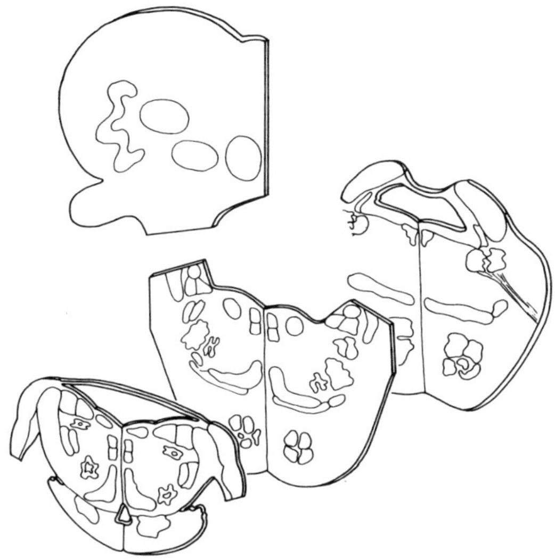

Fig. 5-8. This illustration is a companion to that shown in Fig. 5-7 and may be used to outline the trajectory of fibers through lesions outlined thereon.

TRACT/FIBERS	RELATIONSHIP TO LESION	
	CELLS OF ORIGIN	TERMINATION

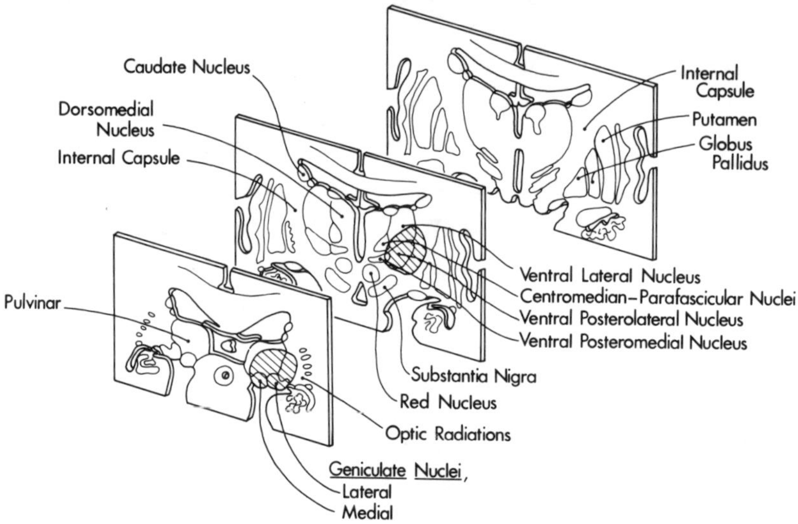

Fig. 6-1. THALAMIC SYNDROME (DÉJÉRINE-ROUSSY SYNDROME): This syndrome is characterized by intractable persistent pain which is usually poorly localized. Additional signs may also be present depending on the degree of involvement of surrounding structures. The thalamic syndrome most frequently results from an occlusion of the thalamogeniculate branch of the posterior cerebral artery.

DEFICIT	ASSOCIATED STRUCTURES
A. Contralateral hemihypalgesia, and intense pain (burning sensation)	A. Ventral posterolateral thalamic nucleus and adjacent white matter
B. Contralateral hemiparesis, Babinski sign, hyperreflexia	B. Corticospinal fibers in posterior of internal capsule
C. Homonymous hemianopsia	C. Lateral geniculate nucleus

COMMENT: Intense "thalamic pain" is the cardinal sign of the thalamic syndrome. Bizzare paresthesias, such as a sensation of ants crawling on the skin, may also be experienced. The thalamogeniculate artery serves most of the structures included in the lesion.

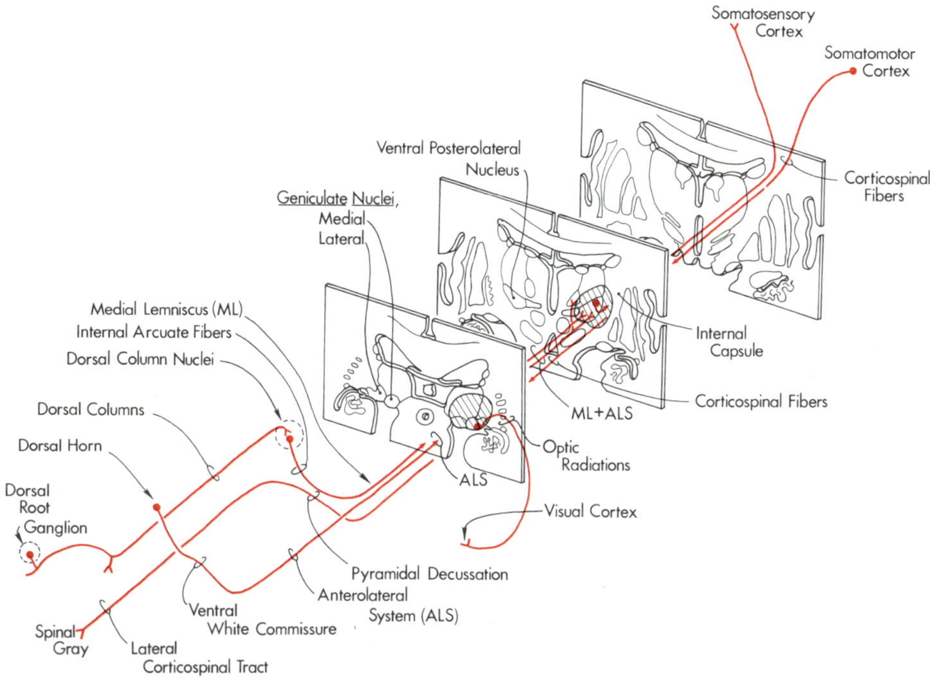

Fig. 6-2. Trajectory of fibers and locations of cells responsible for the symptoms seen in the thalamic syndrome.

	RELATIONSHIP TO LESION	
TRACT/FIBERS	CELLS OF ORIGIN	TERMINATION
A. Ventral posterolateral thalamic nucleus in lesion	Contralateral dorsal horn (via anterolateral system	Ipsilateral somatosensory cortex
B. Corticospinal fibers in the posterior limb of internal capsule	Ipsilateral somatomotor cortex	Contralateral spinal gray
C. Lateral geniculate nucleus in lesion	Ganglion cells of retina bilaterally	Ipsilateral visual cortex

COMMENT: Although the VPL of thalamus also receives position and vibratory sense and discriminative touch from the contralateral side of the body via the dorsal column-medial lemniscus system (see above drawing), loss of these modalities is not a common feature of the thalamic syndrome. Involvement of the medial geniculate may produce a slight dimunition of hearing on the ipsilateral side. The intense unrelenting pain characteristic of the thalamic syndrome is related not only to the destruction of nerve tissue but also to the fact that the lesion is highly irritating to adjacent areas of the thalamus and the surrounding white matter.

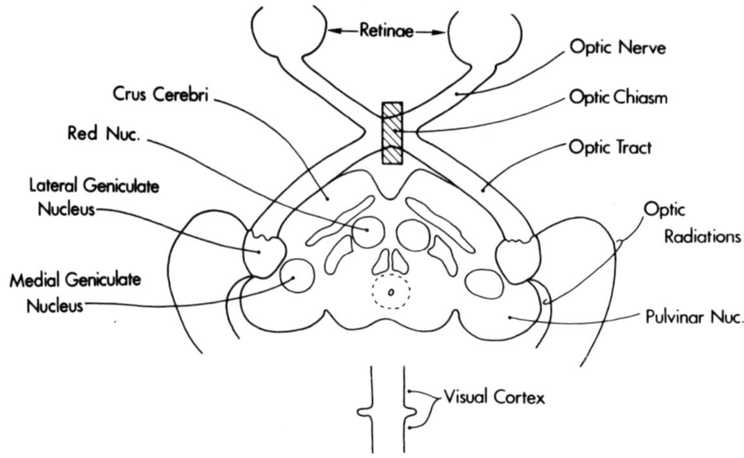

Fig. 6-3. LESION OF THE OPTIC CHIASM (CROSSING FIBERS): Damage to the crossing fibers of the optic chiasm may result from tumors of the pituitary (i.e., adenoma) or craniopharyngiomas. Lesions of the pituitary will produce neuroendocrine problems of varying types and severity. Only visual problems are shown here.

DEFICIT	ASSOCIATED STRUCTURES
A. Bitemporal heteronymous hemianopsia	A. Central regions of the optic chiasm (crossing fibers)

COMMENT: Since the ganglion cells of each eye project into the pretectal area (nucleus) and this group of cells projects bilaterally to the Edinger-Westphal nucleus, a lesion of the crossing fibers will not cause a loss of the pupillary light reflex. Such a loss could be demonstrated if light is shown as a focused source on small areas of temporal versus nasal retinae.

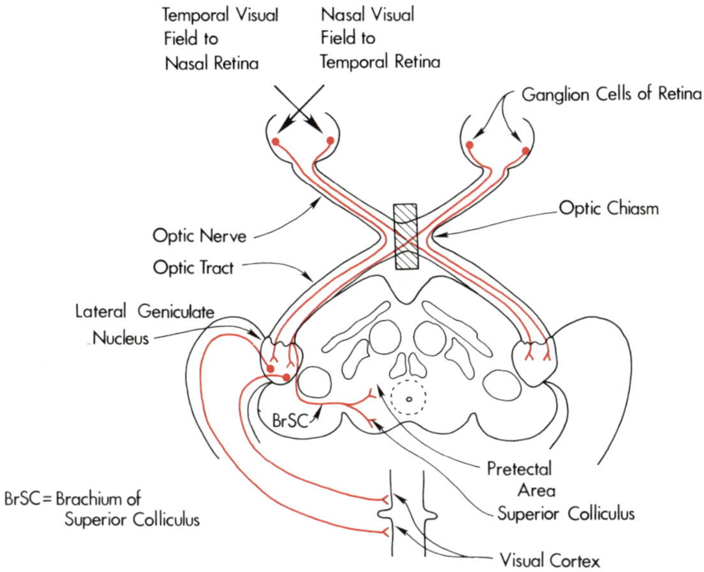

Fig. 6-4. Trajectory of fibers involved in a lesion of the crossing fibers of the optic chiasm.

TRACT/FIBERS	RELATIONSHIP TO LESION	
	CELLS OF ORIGIN	TERMINATION
A. Retinogeniculate fibers in the chiasm	Ganglion cells in the nasal areas of retina bilaterally	Bilateral lateral geniculate nuclei (vision), bilateral pretectal area (pupillary light reflex pathway), and superior colliculus

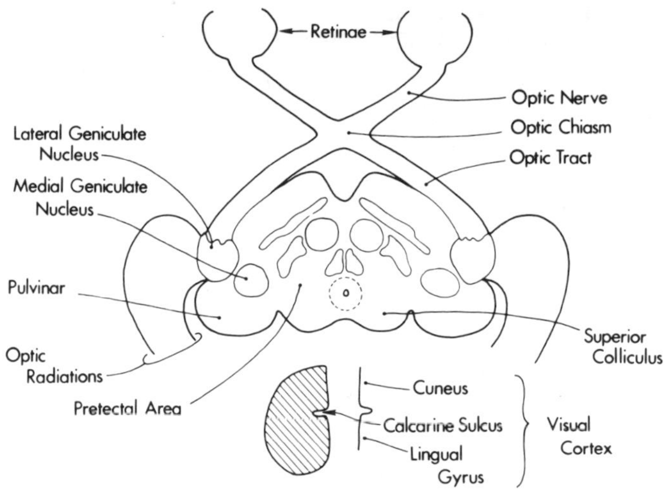

Fig. 6-5. LESION OF THE VISUAL CORTEX: Destruction of the visual cortex may follow an occlusion of distal branches of the posterior cerebral artery. The calcarine branch of the posterior cerebral artery serves the visual cortex.

DEFICIT	ASSOCIATED STRUCTURES
A. Right homonymous hemianopsia	A. Left visual cortex, area 17
B. Loss of upward gaze	B. Corticotectal projections form occipital cortex (areas 18,19) to superior colliculus

COMMENT: Macular vision may be spared since the cortical region which receives this input is at the caudal extremity of the calcarine sulcus and receives additional blood supply by terminal branches of the middle cerebral artery. Thrombosis of the distal portions of the posterior cerebral artery may affect visual cortex (#17) and the surrounding cortical areas (#18,19) and other occipital cortical regions. Alexia (inability to recognize printed or written word) and visual agnosia (failure of object recognition) may also be seen following occipital cortical lesions.

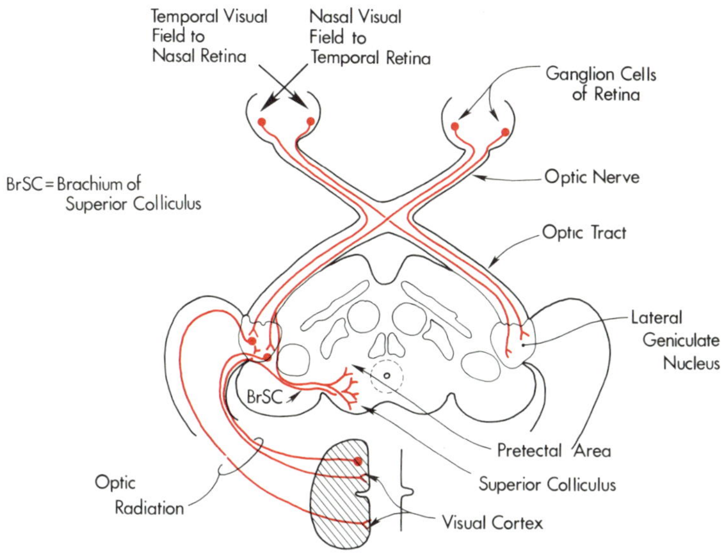

Fig. 6-6. Trajectory of fibers and location of neurons responsible for the symptoms seen in a lesion of the visual cortex.

	RELATIONSHIP TO LESION	
TRACT/FIBERS	CELLS OF ORIGIN	TERMINATION
A. Geniculocalcarine fibers in lesion, occipital cortex	Ipsilateral lateral geniculate nucleus	Ipsilateral visual cortex (in lesion)
B. Cells of origin of corticotectal fibers	Ipsilateral visual cortex (#17) and areas #18, #19 (in lesion)	Ipsilateral superior colliculus, and pretectal area.

COMMENT: In addition to projections into the superior colliculus and pretectal area, the visual cortex and areas 18 and 19 also project to the pons (corticopontine fibers), the reticular formation (corticoreticular fibers) and the pulvinar nucleus of the thalamus. The visual cortex also projects into the ipsilateral lateral geniculate body.

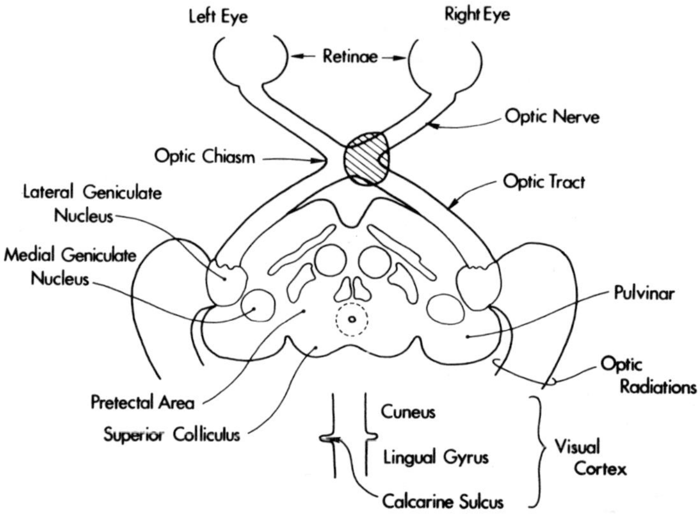

Fig. 6-7. PITUITARY ADENOMA. In this example a tumor of the pituitary has compromised the optic chiasm (crossing fibers) plus the entire right optic nerve just rostral to the chiasm and the right optic tract just caudal to the chiasm.

DEFICIT	ASSOCIATED STRUCTURES
A.	A. Retinal ganglion cell projections to lateral geniculate body (visual)
B.	B. Retinal ganglion cell projections to pretectal nuclei (reflex)

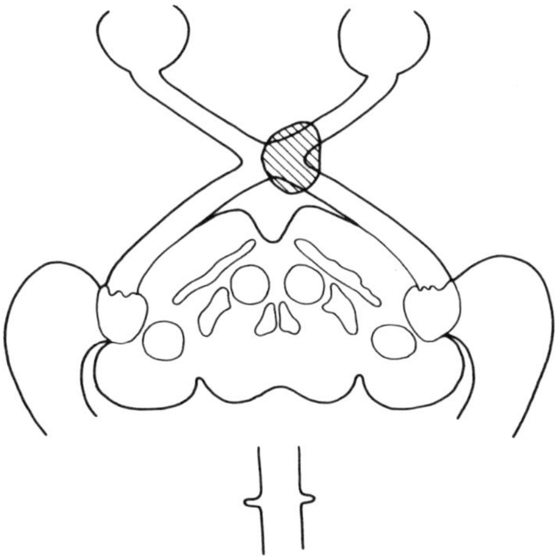

Fig. 6-8. Trajectory of fibers responsible for the symptoms seen in a lesion of the crossing fibers in the optic chiasm as well as the optic nerve and optic tract on the right side.

TRACT/FIBERS	RELATIONSHIP TO LESION CELLS OF ORIGIN	TERMINATION
A.		
B.		

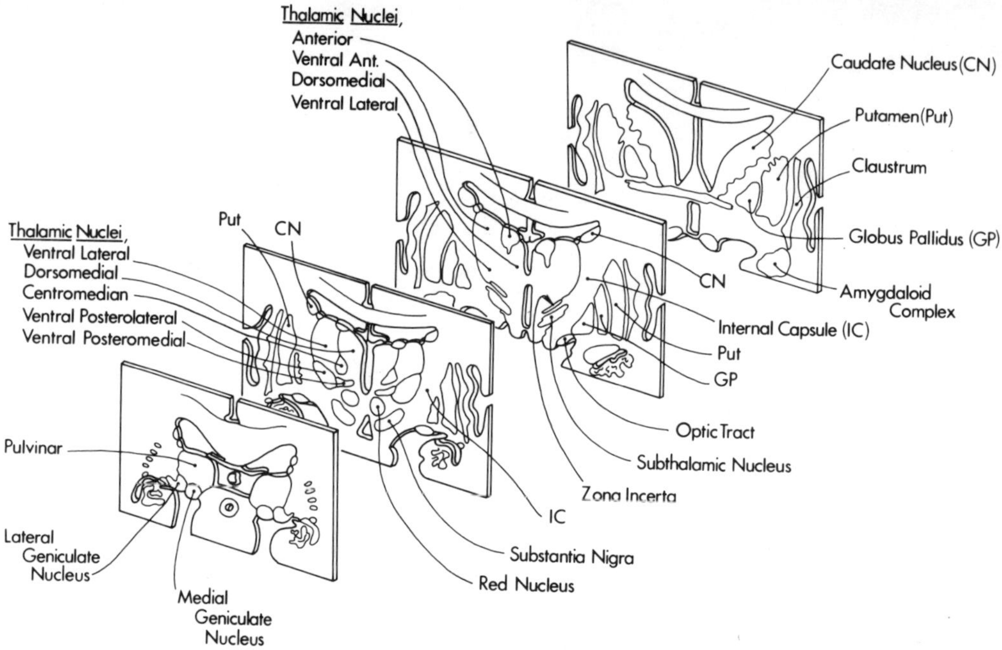

Fig. 6-9. BASIC CONNECTIONS OF THE BASAL GANGLIA: This illustration does not contain a lesion but is an overview of the connections of the basal ganglia for the example cases to follow (see Figs. 6-13 to 6-18).

As usually defined, the basal ganglia consist of the corpus striatum and the amygdaloid nuclear complex; only connections of the corpus striatum are considered here. The corpus striatum is divided into the neostriatum (caudate nucleus + putamen) and the paleostriatum (globus pallidus). The amygdaloid nuclear complex is sometimes referred to as the archistriatum The claustrum, although separated from the putamen by the thin external capsule, is probably more closely related to the cerebral cortex. In a broader context, the term basal ganglia has been used to designate, in addition to the above defined structures, other nuclear groups which are functionally related to the corpus striatum, these being the substantia nigra and the subthalamic nucleus.

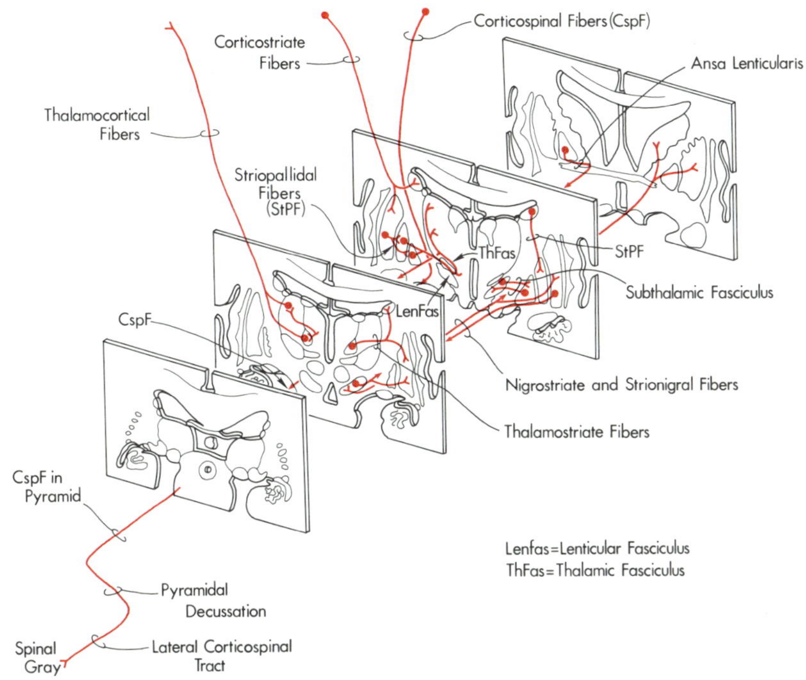

Fig. 6-10. Principal afferent and efferent connections of the corpus striatum, substantia nigra, and subthalamic nucleus. In general the neostriatum (caudate nucleus + putamen) is the afferent receiving portion of the corpus striatum and the paleostriatum (globus pallidus) is the efferent projecting portion.

Most areas of cerebral cortex project into the neostriatum as corticostriate fibers. The caudate nucleus and putamen in turn project, as striopallidal fibers, into both inner and outer segments of the globus pallidus. Cells of the globus pallidus give rise to two main efferent bundles. The first, the ansa lenticularis (ALen) originates from slightly more rostral levels and courses medially and caudally toward Forel's field. The second bundle is the lenticular fasciculus (LenFas). It originates from slightly more caudal portions of the globus pallidus, traverses the posterior limb of the internal capsule and courses between the subthalamic nucleus and zona incerta to enter Forel's field. Within Forel's field the ALen and LenFas enter the thalamic fasciculus and are subsequently distributed to several nuclei of the dorsal thalamus (VA, VL, CM). Cerebellothalamic fibers, originating in the contralateral cerebellar nuclei (see Fig. 5-2) also course into these nuclei through the thalamic fasciculus. Thalamostriate fibers, primarily from the centromedian-parafascicular complex and other intralaminar nuclei, also represent an important source of neostriatial afferents. The subthalamic nucleus is reciprocally connected with the globus pallidus by way of the subthalamic fasciculus. The substantia nigra is interconnected with the corpus striatum by way of strionigral and nigrostriatal fibers. Those thalamic nuclei which receive pallidal (and cerebellar) input project to the cerebral cortex through thalamocortical fibers. Corticospinal fibers, although included on this illustration, are not considered as part of the afferent/efferent connections of the corpus striatum. They are shown to illustrate the point that the somatomotor expression of basal ganglia dysfunction will follow the trajectory of these fibers.

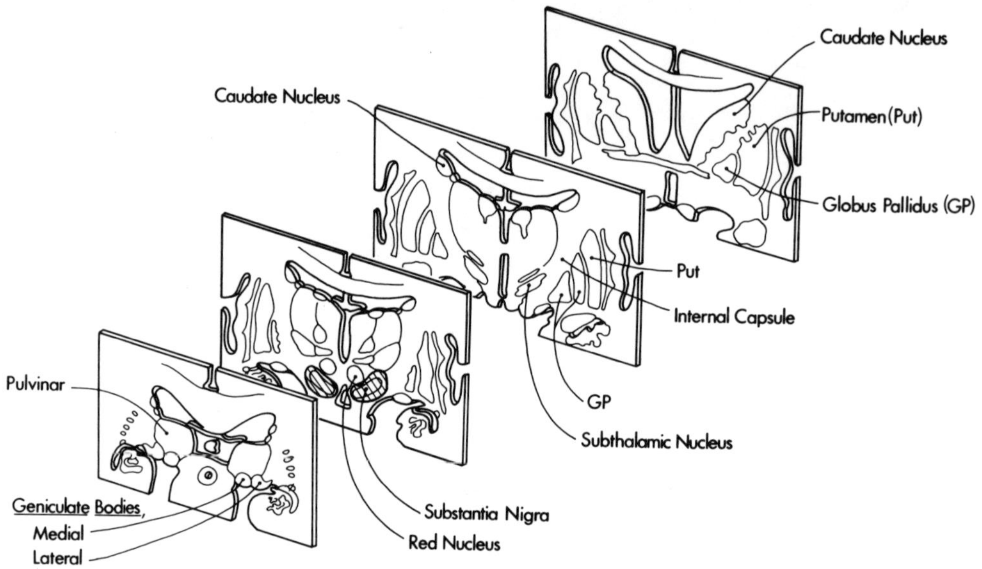

Fig. 6-11. **PARKINSON'S DISEASE, LESIONS OF THE SUBSTANTIA NIGRA:** This disease may be the result of arteriosclerosis, idiopathic in origin, or be seen following an attack of encephalitis lethargica. Idiopathic parkinsonism is probably the most common type. The most prominent area damaged in the substantia nigra.

DEFICIT

A. Tremor (pill-rolling), cog wheel (muscle) rigidity, festinating gait, stooped posture, expressionless face, and bradykinesia

ASSOCIATED STRUCTURES

A. Substantia nigra; cell loss in this nucleus, loss of nigral efferents and ineffective nigral afferents

COMMENT: The parkinsonian tremor is frequently referred to as a 'resting tremor' since it is most evident at rest and may diminish or temporarily disappear during volutional movement. Atrophy and cell loss is sometimes seen in the globus pallidus and in some areas of the cerebral cortex in this disease. The festinating gait seen in Parkinson patients is characterized as rapid, quick and accelerated.

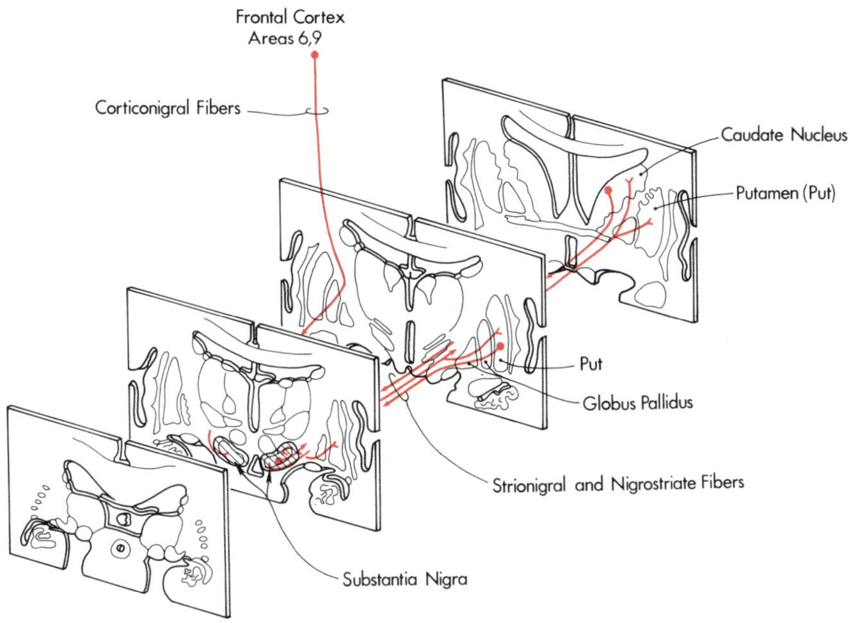

Fig. 6-12. Trajectory of fibers responsible for the symptoms seen in a lesion of the substantia nigra (Parkinson's Disease).

TRACT/FIBERS	RELATIONSHIP TO LESION: CELLS OF ORIGIN	TERMINATION
A. Substantia nigra in the lesion		
-Afferents	Ipsilateral frontal cortex	Ipsilateral substantia nigra in lesion
	Ipsilateral neostriatum	Strionigral terminals in lesion
-Efferents	Ipsilateral substantia nigra in lesion	Ipsilateral caudate nucleus and putamen

COMMENT: The substantia nigra also projects to the subthalamic, amygdaloid and thalamic nuclei and to the superior colliculus. It also receives input from the amygdaloid complex and the raphe nuclei. There is a marked decrease, or complete absence, of dopamine in the substantia nigra and portions of the neostriatum in parkinsonism. This lack of dopamine (which inhibits the firing of striatal neurons) may produce a release phenomenon which accounts for the marked increase in motor activity seen in this disease.

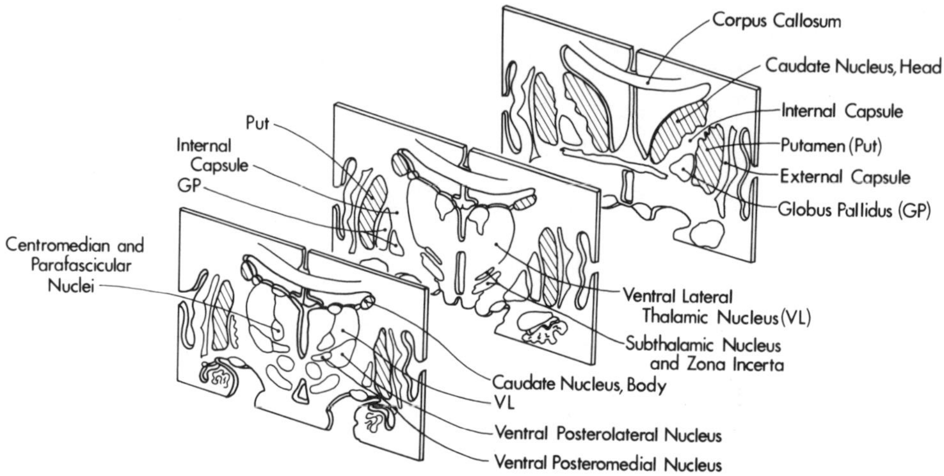

Fig. 6-13. **HUNTINGTON'S CHOREA, NEURONAL LOSS IN THE CAUDATE NUCLEUS AND PUTAMEN:** This is an inherited disease (autosomal dominant trait) which becomes clinically evident during adult life. It is characterized by severe cell loss and atrophy in the neostriatum.

DEFICIT

A. Choreiform movements of extremities, face, tongue, lips and head, unsteady jerky gait

ASSOCIATED STRUCTURES

A. Degenerative changes in the neostriatum (caudate nucleus and putamen)

COMMENT: The choreiform movements may appear before or after the onset of dementia, or they may both appear at about the same time. Although not as marked as in the striatum, atrophy, cell loss and gliosis may also be present in the cerebral cortex particularly the frontal lobes. The dementia seen in Huntington's chorea is primarily related to the cell loss and gliosis in the frontal cortex. The three main characteristics of Huntington's chorea are; 1) it is an autosomal dominant inherited disease, 2) chorea and dementia occur in the same patient and, 3) the disease usually appears during adult life. There are, however, juvenile forms of Huntington's chorea.

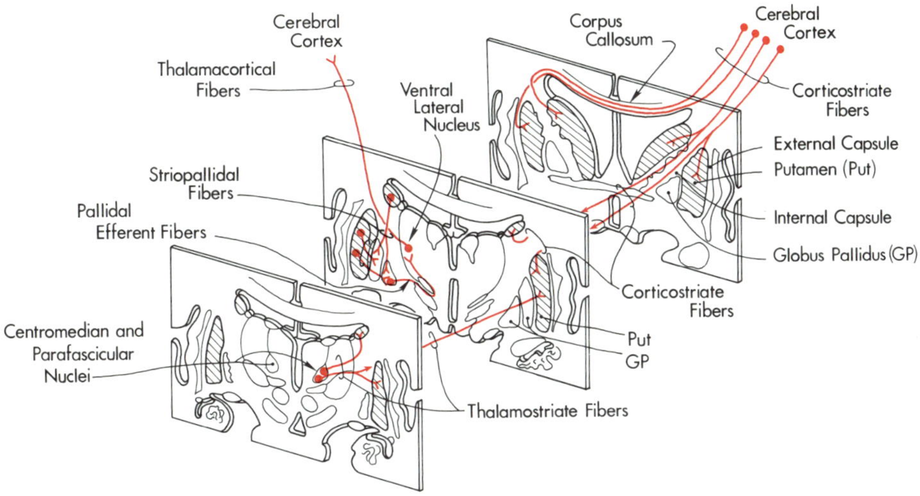

Fig. 6-14. Trajectory of fibers responsible for the motor symptoms seen in Huntington's chorea (cell loss, atrophy and gliosis of the caudate nucleus and putamen).

	RELATIONSHIP OF LESION	
TRACT/FIBERS	CELLS OF ORIGIN	TERMINATION
A. Caudate nucleus, putamen in lesion bilaterally		
-Afferents	Bilateral cerebral cortex	Neostriatum in lesion bilaterally
	Ipsilateral thalamic nuclei	Ipsilateral neostriatum in lesion
-Efferents	Cells in ipsilateral neostriatum in lesion	Ipsilateral globus pallidus

COMMENT: A loss of control over the muscles of respiration and speech may produce marked difficulty in verbal expression. Studies on patients with Huntington's chorea indicate a significant decrease in gamma-aminobutyric acid containing neurons in the corpus striatum.

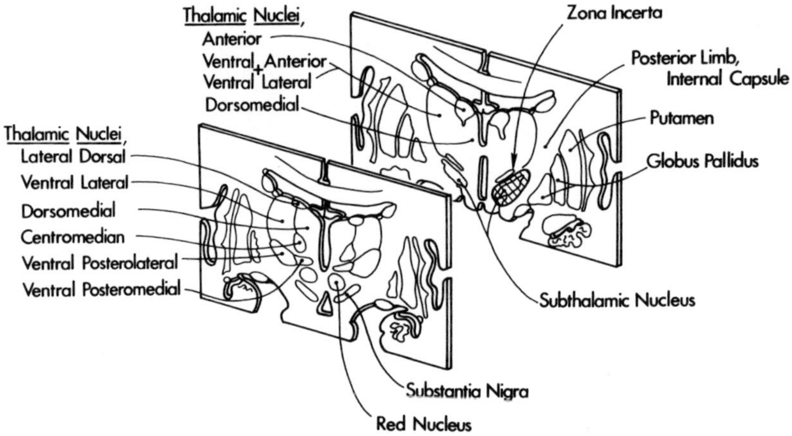

Fig. 6-15. HEMIBALLISM, LESION OF THE SUBTHALAMIC NUCLEUS: This is usually the result of a hemorrhage or occlusion of small vessels supplying the subthalamic nucleus or its immediate environs. Tumors located in the subthalamic area may also produce hemiballism but this is a relatively rare causative factor.

DEFICIT	ASSOCIATED STRUCTURES
A. Contralateral hemiballism, violent flailing movements of extremities (primarily the upper)	A. Subthalamic nucleus and its main connections

COMMENT: The wild movements seen in hemiballism are made worse by stress, partially relieved by relaxation, constantly present in the awake state, and usually absent when the patient is asleep.

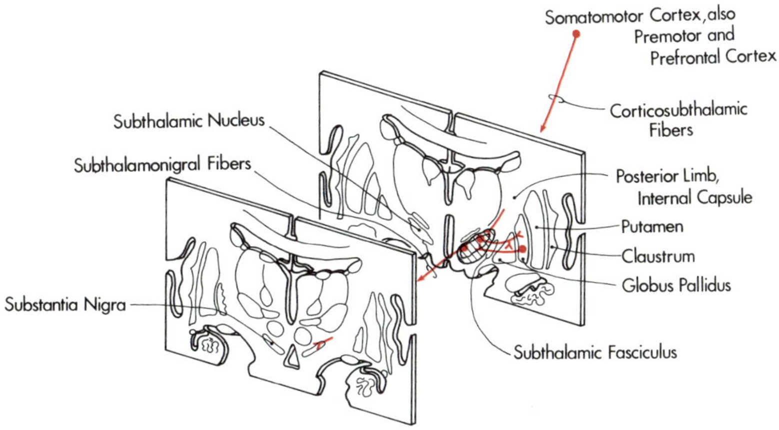

Fig. 6-16. Trajectory of fibers responsible for the symptoms seen in a lesion of the subthalamic nucleus producing hemiballism.

TRACT/FIBERS	RELATIONSHIP TO LESION: CELLS OF ORIGIN	TERMINATION
A. Subthalamic nucleus in lesion		
-Afferents	Ipsilateral somatomotor, prefrontal and premotor cortices	Ipsilateral subthalamic nucleus in lesion
	Ipsilateral globus pallidus	Ipsilateral subthalamic nucleus in lesion
-Efferents	Ipsilateral subthalamic nucleus in lesion	Ipsilateral globus pallidus and substantia nigra

COMMENT: The hemiballism characteristic of a lesion in the subthalamus is seen on the side of the body contralateral to the lesion. Damage to the subthalamic nucleus apparently removes a powerful inhibitory influence on the globus pallidus. Since the latter is the primary efferent pathway of the corpus striatum (via the ansa lenticularis and lenticular fasciculi) the removal of this inhibitory influence results in uncontrolled discharges through the pallidothalamic-thalamocortical-corticospinal circuit. The results are violent forceful movements on the contralateral side of the body. Due to the decussation of corticospinal fibers, the motor deficits are seen contralateral to the lesion (see Fig. 6-10).

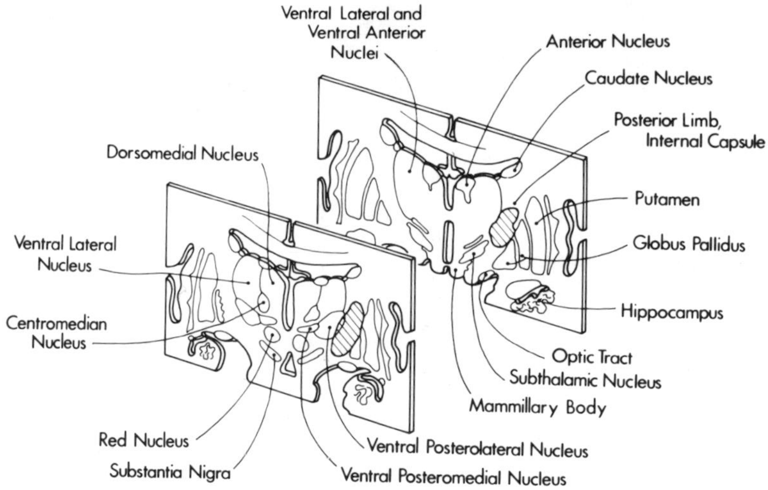

Fig. 6-17. LESION IN THE POSTERIOR LIMB OF THE INTERNAL CAPSULE: Small lesions in the internal capsule may be the result of small hemorrhages. Although the anterior choroidal artery provides a significant blood supply to the internal capsule total occlusion of this vessel is rare.

DEFICIT	ASSOCIATED STRUCTURES
A. Contralateral hemiparesis, Babinski sign	A. Corticospinal fibers in internal capsule
B. Contralateral paralysis of lower facial muscles	B. Corticobulbar fibers in internal capsule
C. Contralateral diminution or loss of pain and temperature sensation (body and face), position and vibratory sense and discriminitive touch	C. Interruption of thalamocortical fibers from VPM and VPL to somatosensory cortex

COMMENT: A lesion in this location will characteristically produce motor deficits. In addition there may also be a weakness of the tongue contralaterally (deviation away from the side of the lesion on protrusion) and a deviation of the uvula to the side of the lesion on phonation. Sensory losses, as included here, may be more variable depending on the extent of the lesion. Such signs may be seen as diminution or losses of the respective sensations, paresthesias, hyperesthesias, or a constant discomfort similar to the thalamic syndrome (see Fig. 6-1).

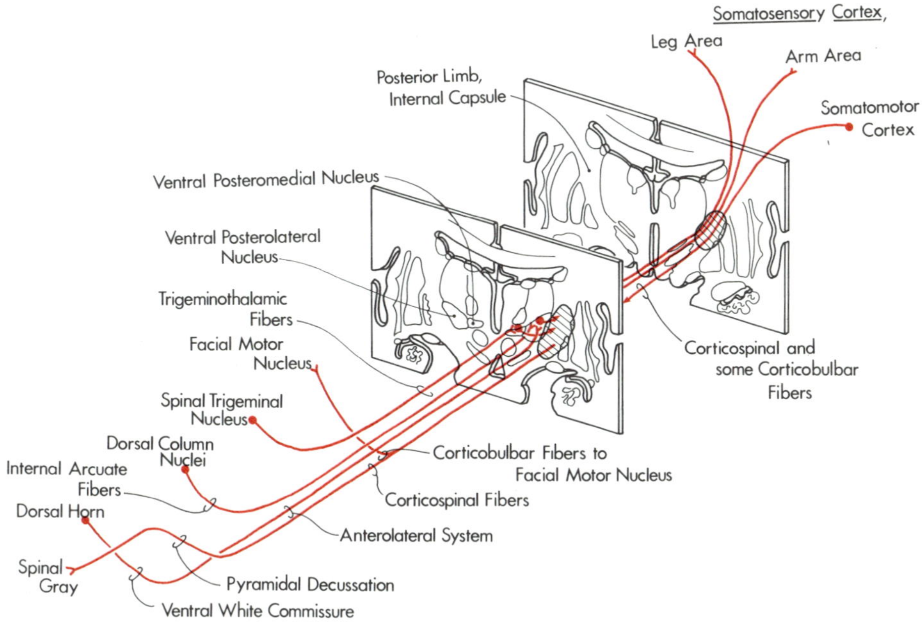

Fig. 6-18. Trajectory of fibers responsible for the symptoms seen in a lesion of the posterior limb of the internal capsule.

	RELATIONSHIP TO LESION	
TRACT/FIBERS	CELLS OR ORIGIN	TERMINATION
A. Corticospinal fibers	Ipsilateral somatomotor cortex	Contralateral spinal gray
B. Corticobulbar fibers	Ipsilateral face area of somatomotor cortex	Contralateral motor facial nucleus
C. Thalamocortical fibers	Ipsilateral VPM and VPL	Ipsilateral somatosensory cortex

COMMENT: Sensory input to the VPM and VPL originates from the contralateral side of the body. Exteroceptive data (pain and temperature sensations) to VPM is relayed via cells of the contralateral spinal trigeminal nucleus (as ventral trigeminothalamic fibers) while the same type of information from the body comes from cells in the contralateral dorsal horn through the anterolateral system to the VPL. Proprioceptive information (position and vibratory sense, touch), is relayed by cells of the contralateral dorsal column nuclei to the VPL via the medial lemniscus and bilaterally to the VPM by cells of the chief sensory nucleus. Although corticospinal and corticobulbar fibers are diagrammatically represented here as one fiber, it is well known that they originate from body and face areas, respectively, of the somatomotor cortex.

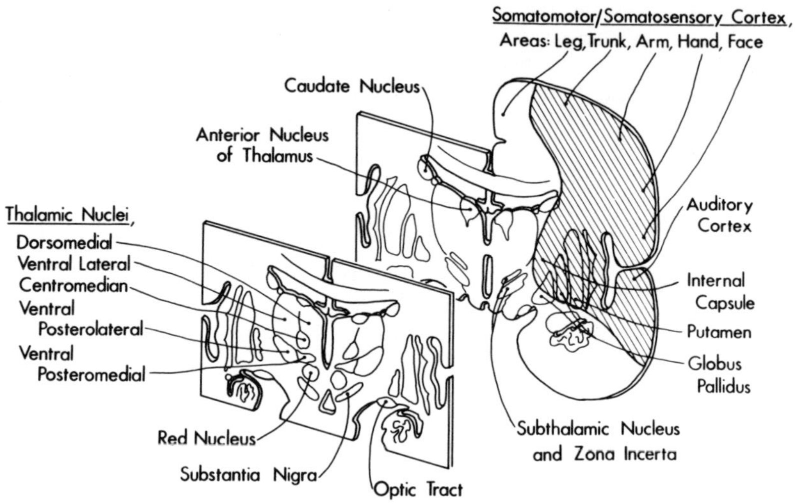

Fig. 6-19. OCCLUSION OF THE MIDDLE CEREBRAL ARTERY: Occlusion of the middle cerebral artery may be caused by either thrombosis or embolus and may occur proximally (close to its origin from the internal carotid), or distally (involving primarily cortical branches). The example shown here is proximal.

DEFICIT	ASSOCIATED STRUCTURES
A. Contralateral hemiplegia of lower face, trunk, upper and lower extremities, Babinski sign	A. Somatomotor cortex and corticospinal and corticobulbar fibers in internal capsule
B. Contralateral hemianesthesia (or hemihypesthesia) of face, trunk, upper and lower extremities	B. Somatosensory cortex and thalamocortical fibers from VPM/VPL in internal capsule
C. Homonymous hemianopsia	C. Geniculocalcarine fibers looping through temporal and parietal lobes

COMMENT: The symptoms seen following blockage of the middle cerebral artery vary widely depending on the location of the occlusion. Losses are most severe when the occlusion is proximal since this will affect wide areas of cortex, most of the internal capsule, parts of the basal ganglia and the optic radiations as they course through the white matter of temporal and parietal lobes.

Dominant hemisphere: In addition to the above deficits, infarction of the dominant hemisphere will result in global aphasia, right-left disorientation, apraxia (ideational and ideomotor), finger agnosia, agraphia, and acalculia.

Non-dominant hemisphere: In addition to the above deficits, infarction of the non-dominant hemisphere will result in neglect of the affected side, inability to recognize deficits on the affected side, apraxia (constructional, dressing), and difficulty in recognizing faces.

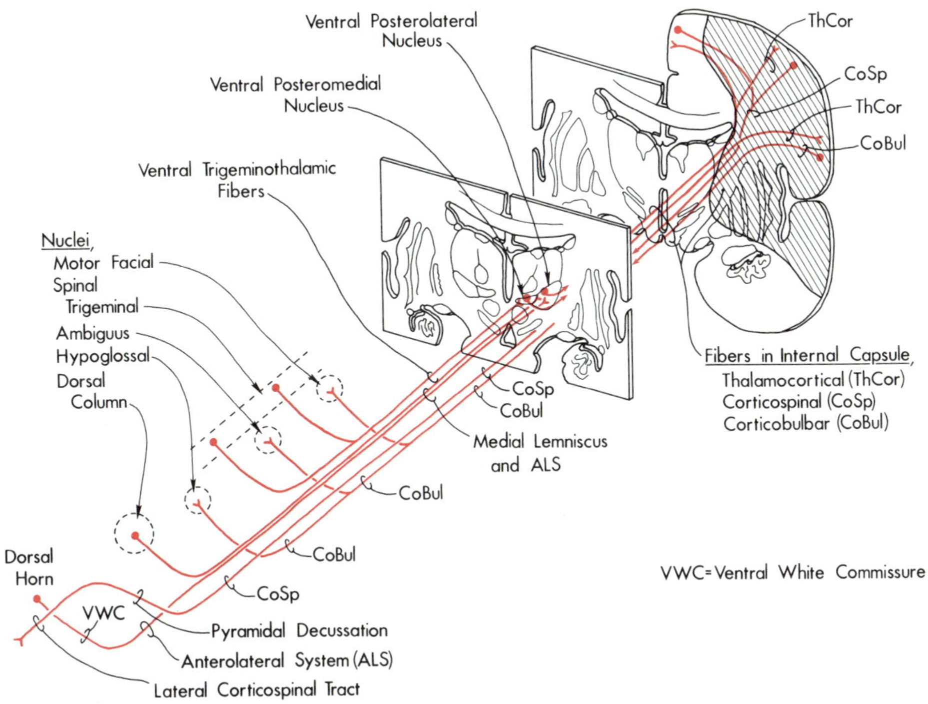

Fig. 6-20. Trajectory of fibers responsible for the motor, sensory, and visual problems related to an occlusion of the proximal middle cerebral artery.

	RELATIONSHIP TO LESION	
TRACT/FIBERS	CELLS OF ORIGIN	TERMINATION
A. Corticospinal fibers	Somatomotor cortex in lesion and fibers in internal capsule	Contralateral spinal gray
Corticobulbar fibers	Somatomotor cortex in lesion and fibers in internal capsule	Portions of contralateral facial and hypoglossal nuclei, nucleus ambiguus
B. Thalamocortical fibers	Ipsilateral VPM and VPL	Ipsilateral somatosensory cortex in lesion
C. Geniculocalcarine (visual) fibers	Ipsilateral lateral geniculate nucleus (see Figs. 6-4, 6-6)	Ipsilateral visual cortex (see Figs. 6-4, 6-6)

COMMENT: Exteroceptive and proprioceptive input to the VPM and VPL nuclei of the thalamus are via the dorsal column-medial lemniscus system and the anterolateral system (for the body) and through trigeminothalamic fibers (for the head); only ventral trigeminothalamic fibers are shown. Occlusion of distal branches will produce variations on those described in Fig. 6-19. For example, blockage of the Rolandic branch will result in only motor and sensory losses with the leg largely spared. Occlusion of parietal banches will result in an inferior homonymous quadrantanopsia while involvement of temporal branches will produce a superior homonymous quadrantanopsia; other cortical signs will accompany these characteristic motor, sensory, and visual deficits. Although auditory cortex is usually involved, hearing losses are not an obvious sign.

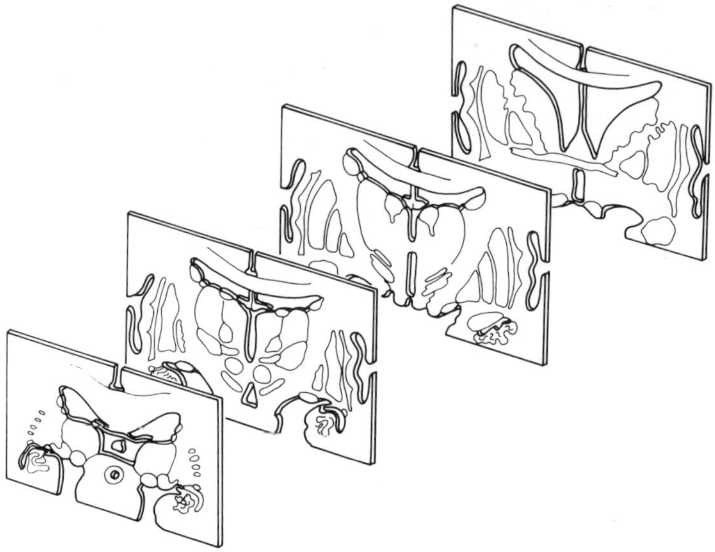

Fig. 6-21. Blank master drawing of representative levels through the thalamus, diencephalon, basal ganglia, and internal capsule. This illustration can be used to outline lesions of the user's choice and to correlate the subsequent deficits with particular structures.

<u>DEFICIT</u>	<u>ASSOCIATED STRUCTURES</u>

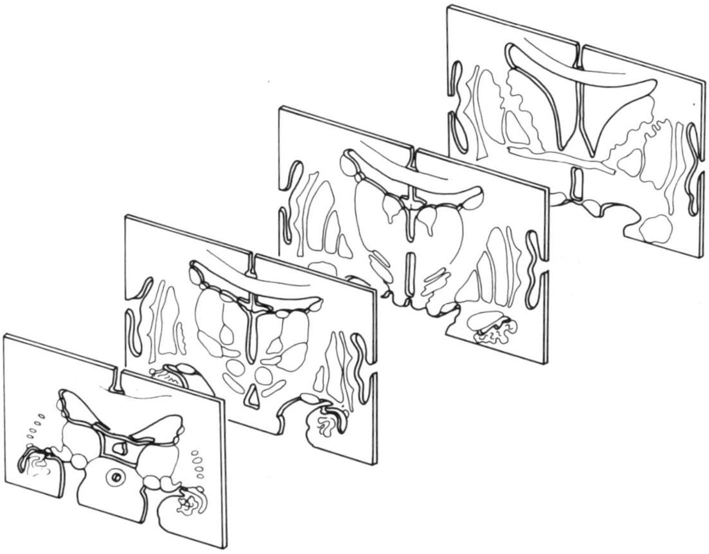

Fig. 6-22. This illustration is the companion to Fig. 6-21 and may be used to outline the trajectory of fibers passing through lesions outlined thereon.

TRACT/FIBERS	RELATIONSHIP TO LESION	
	CELLS OF ORIGIN	TERMINATION

SOURCES AND SUGGESTED READINGS

Angevine, J.B., C.W. Cotman: Principles of Neuroanatomy. Oxford University Press, New York, 1981.

Bannister, R.: Brain's Clinical Neurology, 5th Edition. Oxford University Press, New York, 1978.

Barr, M.L., J.A. Kiernan: The Human Nervous System, An Anatomical Viewpoint, 4th Edition. Harper & Row, Philadelphia, 1983.

Bertram, E.G.M., K.L. Moore: An Atlas of the Human Brain and Spinal Cord. Williams & Wilkins, Baltimore, 1982.

Bossy, J.: Atlas of Neuroanatomy and Special Sense Organs. W.B. Saunders Company, Philadelphia, 1970.

Brodal, A.: Neurological Anatomy in Relation to Clinical Medicine, 3rd Edition. Oxford University Press, New York, 1981.

Carpenter, M.B., J. Sutin: Human Neuroanatomy, 8th Edition. Williams & Wilkins, Baltimore, 1983.

Clemente, C.D.: Anatomy, A Regional Atlas of the Human Body, 2nd Edition. Urban & Schwarzenberg, Baltimore, 1981.

Collins, R.D.: Illustrated Manual of Neurologic Diagnosis, 2nd Edition. J.B. Lippincott, Philadelphhia, 1982.

Crosby, E.C., T. Humphrey, E.W. Lauer: Correlative Anatomy of the Nervous System. Macmillan, New York, 1962.

Curtis, B.A., S. Jacobson, E.M. Marcus: An Introduction to the Neurosciences. W.B. Saunders Company, Philadelphia, 1972.

Daube, J.R., B.A. Sandok, T.J. Reagan, B.F. Westmoreland: Medical Neurosciences, An Approach to Anatomy, Pathology, and Physiology by Systems and Levels. Little, Brown, and Company, Boston, 1978.

DeArmond, S.J., M.M. Fusco, M.M. Dewey: A Photographic Atlas, Structure of the Human Brain, 2nd Edition. Oxford University Press, New York, 1976.

deGroot, J.: Correlative Neuroanatomy of Computed Tomography and Magnetic Resonance Imaging. Lea & Febiger, Philadelphia, 1984.

Dublin, A.B., W.B. Dublin: Atlas of Neuroanatomy with Radiologic Correlation and Pathologic Illustration. Warren H. Green, Inc., St. Louis, 1982.

Eliasson, S.G., A.L. Prensky, W.B. Hardin, Jr.: Neurological Pathophysiology, 2nd Edition. Oxford University Press, New York, 1978.

Farmer, T.W. (Ed.): Pediatric Neurology, 2nd Edition. Harper & Row, New York, 1975.

Ferner, H. (Ed.): Eduard Pernkopf Atlas of Topographical and Applied Human Anatomy, 2nd Revised Edition. Volume I, Head and Neck. Urban & Schwarzenberg, Baltimore, 1980.

Fix, J.D., C.S. Punte: Atlas of the Human Brain Stem and Spinal Cord. University Park Press, Baltimore, 1981.

Ford, D.H., J. Illari, J.P. Schade: Atlas of the Human Brain, 3rd Edition. Elsevier/North Holland, Amsterdam and New York, 1978.

Ganong, W.F.: The Nervous System. Lange Medical Publications, Los Altos, 1977.

Gilman, S., S.S. Winans: Manter and Gatz's Essential of Clinical Neuroanatomy and Neurophysiology, 6th Edition. F.A. Davis Company, Philadelphia, 1982.

Gilman, S., J.R. Bloedel, R. Lechtenberg: Disorders of the Cerebellum. F.A. Davis Company, Philadelphia, 1981.

Gluhbegovic, N., T.H. Williams: The Human Brain, A Photographic Guide. Harper & Row, Hagerstown, 1980.

Haines, D.E.: Neuroanatomy, An Atlas of Structures, Sections, and Systems. Urban & Schwarzenberg, Baltimore, 1983.

Hamilton, W.J., H.W. Mossman: Human Embryology, 4th Edition. W. Heffer & Sons, Ltd., Cambridge and Williams & Wilkins, Baltimore, 1972.

Heimer, L.: The Human Brain and Spinal Cord, Functional Neuroanatomy and Dissection Guide. Springer-Verlag, New York, 1983.

House, E.L., B. Pansky, A. Siegel: A Systematic Approach to Neuroscience, 3rd Edition. McGraw-Hill Book Company, New York, 1979.

Kandel, E.R., J.H. Schwartz (Eds.): Principles of Neural Science. Elsevier/North-Holland, New York, 1981.

Lewis, A.J.: Mechanisms of Neurological Disease. Little, Brown and Company, Boston, 1976.

Liebman, M.: Neuroanatomy Made Easy and Understandable, 2nd Edition. University Park Press, Baltimore, 1983.

Martinez Martinez, P.F.A.: Neuroanatomy, Development and Structure of the Central Nervous System. W.B. Saunders Company, Philadelphia, 1982.

Matzke, H.A., F.M. Foltz: Synopsis of Neuroanatomy, 4th Edition. Oxford University Press, New York, 1983.

Miller, R.A., E. Burack: Atlas of the Central Nervous System in Man, 3rd Edition. Williams & Wilkins, Baltimore, 1982.

Montemurro, D.G., J.E. Bruni: The Human Brain in Dissection. W.B. Saunders Company, Philadelphia, 1981.

Nieuwenhuys, R., J. Voogd, Chr. van Huijzen: The Central Nervous System, A Synopsis and Atlas. Springer-Verlag, Berlin, 1978.

Noback, C.R., R.J. Demarest: The Human Nervous System, Basic Principles of Neurobiology, 2nd Edition. McGraw-Hill Book Company, New York, 1975.

Nolte, J.: The Human Brain, An Introduction to its Functional Anatomy. C.V. Mosby Company, St. Louis, 1981.

Pansky, B., D.J. Allen: Review of Neuroscience. MacMillan, New York, 1980.

Patton, H.D., J.W. Sundsten, W.E. Crill, P.D. Swanson: Introduction to Basic Neurology. W.B. Saunders Company, Philadelphia, 1976.

Peele, T.L.: The Neuroanatomic Basis For Clinical Neurology, 3rd Edition. McGraw-Hill Book Company, New York, 1977.

Rowland, L.P. (Ed.): Merritt's Textbook of Neurology, 7th Edition. Lea & Febiger, Philadelphia, 1984.

Rosenberg, R.N. (Ed.): Neurology; Volume 5 of The Science and Practice of Clinical Medicine. Grune & Stratton, New York, 1980.

Schneider, R.C., E.A. Kahn, E.C. Crosby, J.A. Taren.: Correlative Neurosurgery, Vols. I and II, 3rd Edition. C.C. Thomas, Springfield, Illinois, 1982.

Schnitzlein, H.N., E.W. Hartley, F.R. Murtagh, L. Grundy, J.T. Fargher: Computed Tomography of the Head and Spine, A Photographic Color Atlas of CT, Gross, and Microscopic Anatomy. Urban & Schwarzenberg, Baltimore, Munich, 1983.

Shepherd, G.M.: Neurobiology. Oxford University Press, New York, 1983.

Singer, M., P.I. Yakovlev: The Human Brain in Sagittal Section. C. C. Thomas, Springfield, 1964.

Snell, R.S.: Clinical Neuroanatomy for Medical Students. Little, Brown and Company, Boston, 1980.

Walton, J.: Introduction to Clinical Neuroscience. Bailliere Tindall, London, 1983.

Warwick, R., P.L. Williams: Gray's Anatomy, 35th British Edition. W.B. Saunders Company, Philadelphia, 1973.

Watson, C.: Basic Human Neuroanatomy, An Introductory Atlas, 2nd Edition. Little, Brown and Company, Boston, 1977.

Werner, J.K.: Neuroscience, A Clinical Perspective. W.B. Saunders Company, Philadelphia, 1980.

Wicke, L.: Atlas of Radiologic Anatomy, 3rd Edition. Urban & Schwarzenberg, Baltimore, 1982.

Willis, W.D., R.G. Grossman: Medical Neurobiology, Neuroanatomical and Neurophysiologic Principles Basic To Clinical Neuroscience, 3rd Edition. C.V. Mosby Company, St. Louis, 1981.

Youmans, J.R. (Ed.): Neurological Surgery, A Comprehensive Reference Guide to the Diagnosis and Management of Neurosurgical Problems, Vols. I-III. W.B. Saunders Company, Philadelphia, 1973.

Zuleger, S., J. Staubesand: Atlas of the Central Nervous System in Sectional Planes. Urban & Schwarzenberg, Baltimore-Munich, 1977.

INDEX

Accommodation, 58
Acoustic neuroma, 28, 30
Acute anterior thoracic cord
  injury, 16, 17
Agnosis, visual, 78
Alcoholic cerebellar
  degeneration, 70, 71
Alexia, 78
Amyotrophic lateral sclerosis, 14
Aneurysm(s), 38, 39, 44, 46, 50,
  62, 78
Ansa lenticularis, 83, 89
Anterolateral system, 2-14, 16-18,
  22, 23, 26, 27, 30, 34, 38-44, 46,
  48, 50, 54, 56, 58-60, 62, 70, 75,
  91, 93
Archistriatum, 82
Artery,
  anterior choroidal, 78, 90
  anterior spinal, 24
  basilar, 38, 39, 42, 46, 54
  calcarine, 78
  middle cerebral, 78, 92, 93
  posterior cerebral, 54, 60, 74, 75,
    78
  posterior communicating, 78
  posterior inferior cerebellar, 26
    34
  posterior spinal, 22
  superior cerebellar, 42, 60
  thalamogeniculate, 74
  vertebral, 24, 38
Astrocytomas, 6, 40, 56, 66, 68
Ataxia, 26, 30, 42, 46, 56, 66, 68-70
Auditory canal, 28, 30
Auditory projections, 29
Autonomic centers, 40

Babinski sign, 2, 12, 14, 16, 38, 54
  74, 90, 92
Bell's palsy, 50
Basal ganglia, 82, 83, 94
Basilar meningitis, 32
Brachium,
  of superior colliculus, 59, 60, 77
    79
Bradykinesia, 84

Cell column,
  intermediolateral, 16, 27
Cerebellar ataxia, 56, 66, 68, 70
Cerebellar peduncles, 42-44, 46, 48,
  54, 56, 57, 60, 62, 64, 66
Cerebellar signs, 30, 42, 56, 66-70
Cerebellopontine angle, 30
Cerebellum,
  anterior lobe of, 23, 70, 71
  flocculonodular lobe, 29, 70
  lesion(s) of, 66, 68, 70
  posterior lobe of, 70
Cerebral aqueduct, 58
Cerebral hemispheres, 12
Chorda tympani branch,
  of facial nerve, 50
Chordoma, 48
Choreiform movements, 86
Claustrum, 82
Colliculus,
  inferior, 29, 54, 58-60, 62
  superior, 54, 56, 58-60, 62, 77, 78-
    80, 85
Commissure,
  ventral white, 4-9, 16-18, 23, 27,
    41, 43, 75, 91, 93
Convergence, loss of, 58
Corpus callosum, 86, 87
Corpus striatum, 82, 87, 89
Cortex,
  areas #18/#19, 59
  auditory, 92, 93
  cerebellar, 26, 27, 31, 66, 67, 69,
    70-72
  cerebral, 31, 67, 82-84, 86, 87
  frontal, 43, 85
  motor, 31, 43
  occipital, 78
  of cerebellum, 68, 71
  prefrontal, 89
  premotor, 89
  somatomotor, 3, 11, 13, 15, 17, 25,
    39, 55, 67, 69, 75, 89, 91-93
  somatosensory, 3, 11, 13, 17, 23, 25,
    27, 41, 43, 45, 55, 57, 75, 91-93
  vermal, 69
  visual, 75-80, 93
Craniopharyngiomas, 76
Crus cerebri, 54, 56, 57, 60, 62, 76
Cuneus, 78, 80

Decomposition of movement, 42
Decussation,
  of corticospinal fibers, 89
  of superior cerebellar peduncle, 43,
    54, 56, 57, 64, 67
  pyramidal, 3, 11, 13, 15, 17, 22, 39,
    55, 67, 83, 91, 93
  ventral tegmental, 67
Degeneration,
  subacute combined of the spinal cord,
    12, 13
Dementia, 86
Diabetes mellitus, 48
Dilated pupil, 56
Disc, intervertebral, 4, 5
Discriminative touch, loss of, 24
Dizziness, 28
Dopamine, 85

Dorsal column(s), 3, 7, 8, 9, 12-14, 16, 75
Dorsal root(s), 2-5, 7, 9, 23
  lateral division, 7, 9, 11, 23
  medial division, 11, 13, 23
Dysarthria, 68, 70
Dysdiadochokinesia, 42, 66
Dysmetria, 30, 66
Dyssynergia, 30, 42

Electromyography, 4, 5
Encephalitis, 84
Enophthalamos, 26, 27
Ependymomas, 68
External capsule, 82, 86, 87
External strabismus, 54, 56
Exteroceptive data, 91
Extremities, 2, 4, 6, 8, 12, 14, 24, 38, 40, 54, 70, 74, 86, 88, 90, 92
Eye,
  tearing, 28
Eye movement,
  deficit in, 58

Fasciculus(i),
  cuneatus, 2, 6, 8, 10-14, 22, 23
  gracilis, 2, 4, 6, 8, 10-14, 18, 22, 23
  lenticular, 83, 89
  medial longitudinal, 27-29, 44, 48, 54, 56, 58, 68, 69
  subthalamic, 83, 89
  thalamic, 43, 67, 83
  uncinate, 69
Festinating gait, 84
Fiber(s), See also Tract(s),
  autonomic, 26
  cerebellar corticonuclear, 69
  cerebellar corticovestibular, 69
  cerebellar nuclear efferent, 67
  cerebellorubral, 56, 60
  cerebellothalamic, 56, 57, 60, 85
  corticobulbar, 50, 54, 55, 62, 90, 91-93
  corticobulbar to facial nucleus, 51
  corticonigral, 85
  corticopontine, 31, 66, 67, 79
  corticoreticular, 79
  corticospinal, 3, 38-40, 46, 48, 54, 55, 62, 66, 67, 71, 74, 75, 83, 89-93
  corticostriate, 83, 87
  corticosubthalamic, 89
  corticotectal, 79
  corticovestibular, 71
  cuneocerebellar, 23
  dorsal spinocerebellar, 23, 31, 71
  dorsal trigeminothalamic, 45
  efferent of cerebellum, 69
  exteroceptive, 3
  extrapyramidal, 12-16, 24,39
  fastigiospinal, 69
  fastigiovestibular, 69
  geniculocalcarine, 79, 92, 93
  internal arcuate, 11, 13, 22, 25, 41, 75, 91
  lateral corticospinal, 10, 15
  lateral vestibulospinal, 69
  medial vestibulospinal, 69
  nigrostriate, 83, 85
  olivocerebellar, 23, 71
  pallidal efferent, 89
  parasympathetic, 62
  pontocerebellar, 66, 71
  primary vestibulocerebellar, 29
  proprioceptive, 3
  reticulospinal, 11, 12, 15
  retinogeniculate, 77
  rubrospinal, 11, 13, 15
  secondary vestibulocerebellar, 29
  spinotectal, 59
  spinothalamic, 9, 10, 13, 16, 26, 40, 42
  strionigral, 83, 85
  striopallidal, 83, 87
  subthalamonigral, 89
  tectospinal, 58, 59
  thalamocortical, 83, 87, 89-93
  thalamostriate, 83, 87
  trigeminothalamic, 23, 41, 56, 58, 60, 91
  ventral spinocerebellar, 71
  ventral trigeminothalamic, 23, 40, 41, 45, 56, 57, 60, 93
  vestibulospinal, 11, 13
Fissure,
  posterolateral, 70
  primary, 70
Foramen,
  intervertebral, 4
  jugular, 32, 33
  stylomastoid, 50
Forel's field, 83
Funiculus,
  lateral, 12

Gamma-aminobutyric acid, 87
Ganglion(ia),
  ciliary, 55, 57, 62
  cochlear, 31
  dorsal root, 2-5, 7, 9, 11, 13, 17, 23, 75
  facial, 23
  geniculate, 31
  glossopharyngeal, 23
  pterygopalatine, 31

spiral (cochlear), 27, 29
superior cervical, 27
trigeminal, 23, 27, 31, 43, 45
vagal, 23
vestibular, 28, 29, 31
Ganglion cells of retina, 59, 75, 77, 79, 80
Geniculate body,
lateral, 54, 56, 58, 59, 62
medial, 54, 56, 58, 60, 62
Glioma(s), 34, 38, 40-42, 48, 60
Gliosis, 6
Globus pallidus, 74, 82-84, 86-90, 92
Gyrus,
lingual, 78, 80
transverse temporal, 29

Headache, 58, 62
Hearing,
diminution of loss of, 26, 28
Hemangioblastomas, 66
Hematoma(s),
extradural, 62
subdural, 62
Hemiballism, 88, 89
Hemihypalgesia, 74
Hemiparesis, 24, 38, 74, 90, 92
Hemiplegia, 10, 24, 38, 39, 54, 92
inferior alternating, 24
middle alternating, 38
superior alternating, 54
Hemorrhage(s), 66, 88, 90
Heteronymous hemianopsia,
bitemporal, 76
Hippocampus, 90
Homonymous hemianopsia, 74
right, 78, 92
Horn(s)
dorsal, 2-10, 12, 14, 16-18, 23, 26, 43, 91, 93
ventral, 2-6, 8-10, 12, 14-18
Huntington's chorea, 86, 87
Hydrosyringomyelia, 6
Hyperreflexia, 2, 38, 74
Hypertonia, 38
Hypesthesia(s), 2, 4, 30, 74, 90, 92
Hyporeflexia, 2, 38, 42
Hypothalamus, 27
Hypotonia, 38, 42

Increased intracranial pressure, 66
Infections, 6, 66
Intention tremor, 42, 56
Intermediate zone, 2, 3, 4, 6, 10, 12, 14-18, 71
Intermediolateral cell column, 16, 27
Internal auditory meatus, 28
Internal capsule, 75, 82-84, 86-94
lesion in, 90, 92
Internal strabismus, 38, 40
Intracranial pressure, 48, 58, 62

Juxtarestiform body, 30, 69-71

Larynx, 27
Lemniscus,
lateral, 28
medial, 11, 22-26, 30, 32, 34, 38-42, 44-46, 48, 50, 54, 56-58, 60, 62, 68, 70, 75, 93
Lenticular fasciculus, 83, 89
Ligament,
posterior longitudinal, 4

Macular vision, 78
Mammillary body, 90
Medial accessory olive, 59
Medulla oblongata, 13, 22, 34, 36, 72
Medulloblastomas, 68
Meningiomas, 2
Meningitis, 44, 50, 62
basilar, 32
Mental changes, 12, 86
Midbrain, 64
Midbrain tegmentum,
glioma, 56
lesion of, 60-61
Miosis, 26, 27
Muscle(s),
atrophy, 5, 14, 42, 44
digastric, 43, 45
extraocular, 38, 54, 56
facial, 28, 45, 51, 55
facial expression, 41
fasciculations, 14
genioglossus, 25
hyoglossus, 25
inferior oblique, 55
inferior rectus, 55, 57
lateral rectus, 39-41
levator palpebrae, 55, 57
masseter, 42
medial rectus, 55, 57
mylohyoid, 43, 45
of extremities, 9, 15
of facial expression, 40, 50, 54, 90, 92-93
of mastication, 42-45, 92-93
of tongue, 24, 25, 28, 54, 55, 90
paresis of facial, 50
somatic, 5
styloglossus, 25
superior oblique, 57
superior rectus, 55, 57
temporal, 42
tensor tympani, 43, 45
tensor veli palatini, 43, 45

tibial, 4
weakness of extremities, 4, 8, 12, 14, 54
Myelosyringosis, 6
Myoclonus, 42

Nausea, 26
Neoplasms, 6,
Neostriatum, 82, 83, 85-87
Nerve(s),
abducens, 38, 39, 41, 43, 46, 48, 69
accessory, 32
cochlear, 27-29
eighth cranial, 28
facial, 30, 31, 41, 42, 46, 50, 51
glossopharyngeal, 26, 32, 33
hypoglossal, 24, 25, 32
intermediate, 50
oculomotor, 57, 60, 62, 63, 69
optic, 59, 76-81
peripheral, 12, 13
spinal, 2, 3, 4, 7, 15
spinal accessory, 32, 33
trigeminal, 22, 23, 30, 31, 40, 42-46
trochlear, 69
vagus, 26, 32, 33
vestibular, 28, 29
Neurofibromas, 2
Nucleus(i),
abducens, 28-30, 38-44, 46, 48, 50, 52, 68, 69
accessory cuneate, 23, 24, 32
ambiguus, 14, 26, 27, 32, 34, 35, 93
amygdaloid, 82, 85
auditory relay, 27
caudate, 74, 82-87, 91, 92
cerebellar, 29, 31, 43, 57, 66-68, 70-72, 83
chief sensory, 30, 31, 38, 40, 42 44-46, 48, 50, 57, 91
cochlear, 26-30, 34
cuneatus, 11, 22-26, 32, 34, 41, 57
dorsal column, 11, 13, 22, 23, 57, 91, 93
dorsal motor vagal, 32
Edinger-Westphal, 54-58, 62, 76
facial, 14, 28, 30, 31, 38, 40-44, 46, 48, 50-52, 54, 55, 91, 93
fastigial, 66, 68, 69
gracilis, 11, 13, 22-26, 32, 41, 57
hypoglossal, 14, 24, 25, 32, 34, 54, 55, 93
inferior olivary, 32, 34, 43, 50, 66, 67, 70
intralaminar of thalamus, 43
lateral cervical, 11
lateral geniculate, 74-80, 82, 84, 93
medial geniculate, 29, 61, 75, 76, 78, 80, 82, 84
mesencephalic, 30, 38, 40, 42-46, 48, 50, 54
motor trigeminal, 30, 42
oculomotor, 28, 29, 54-58, 62, 64, 69
of cerebellum, 29, 43, 57, 66
of Clarke, 14, 71
of lateral lemniscus, 29
pontine, 30, 31, 59, 66, 68-71
pretectal, 76, 77, 79, 80
proprius, 11
pulvinar, 59, 78, 79, 82, 84
raphe, 85
red, 11, 43, 54, 56, 57, 60, 62, 67, 74, 76, 82, 84, 88, 90, 92
reticular, 11, 43
solitary, 22, 24, 26, 28, 30-32, 34, 35, 50
spinal trigeminal, 22-24, 26-28, 31, 32, 34, 35, 40-45, 48, 50, 57, 91, 93
subthalamic, 82-86, 88-90, 92
superior olivary, 28, 29, 48, 50
superior salivatory, 31, 50
thalamic, 31, 43, 57, 69, 75, 78, 79, 84, 85, 87, 88, 90, 92, 93 (see also under Thalamic nuclei)
trapezoid, 28, 29
trigeminal, 14, 30, 38, 40, 42-46, 48, 50
trigeminal motor, 31, 43, 45
trochlear, 29, 54, 56, 58, 62, 64, 69
vestibular, 22, 24, 26-30, 32, 34, 42, 44, 46, 48, 50, 68-71
Nucleus pulposus,
herniated, 4, 5
Numbness, 4
Nystagmus, 26, 30, 66, 68-70

Ocular deficits, 69
Ocular dysmetria, 68
Optic,
chiasm, 59, 76, 77, 80, 81
nerve, 59, 76-81
radiations, 74-76, 78-80, 92
tract, 59, 76-82, 90, 92

Pain, 4, 74
Pain and temperature sensation(s),
loss of, 2, 6, 8, 10, 16, 17, 22, 24, 26, 30, 40, 42, 44, 56, 90, 92
Paleostriatum, 82, 83
Papilledema, 58, 62, 66
Papillomas, 68
Paralysis, 5, 8, 12, 24, 38, 40, 42, 44, 50, 54, 56
Paresthesia(s), 2, 9, 12, 16, 30, 74, 90

of the extremities, 13
Paresis, 5, 14, 16, 24, 40, 54, 56, 74, 90
of upward gaze, 58, 78
Parkinson's disease, 84, 85
Peduncle(s),
inferior cerebellar, 71
middle cerebellar, 30, 31, 42, 46, 66, 70, 71
superior cerebellar, 30, 31, 38, 42-44, 46, 48, 54, 56, 57, 60, 62, 64, 66-68, 70, 71
Periaqueductal gray, 62
Periventricular gray, 44
Pernicious anemia, 12
Pharynx, 27
Phonation, 55
Pinealoma, 58
Pituitary, 76
Pituitary adenoma, 80
Pons, 30, 38, 40, 70, 72, 79
basilar, 38, 40, 42, 46, 48, 70
lesion of, 38, 40, 42, 46
tegmentum, 40, 41
Position and vibratory sense, 2, 9, 75, 90
loss of, 2, 10, 12, 22, 24, 40, 46, 56, 90
Posterior fossa, 32, 42
Pretectal area, 58, 76-80
Proprioception, 39, 91
Ptosis, 26, 27
Pupil, 10, 54
constriction of, 10, 26
Purkinje cells, 69-71
Putamen, 74, 82-90, 92
Pyramid, 22, 24-26, 32, 34, 83

Quadrantanopsia,
superior and inferior, 93

Radicular pain, 2
Reflex bladder, 10
Reflex(es), 16
Achilles, 2, 12
corneal, 30, 42, 44, 45
jaw jerk, 44, 45
patellar, 2, 12
pupillary light, 54, 56, 58, 76-78
sneezing, 44
tendon, 2, 12, 14, 16, 24, 38, 74
Triceps, 2
Restiform body, 22, 23, 26, 28, 31, 32, 66, 68, 70, 71
Reticular formation, 27, 59, 66-69, 79
midbrain, 58, 59
pontine, 59
Retina(e), 76-80
nasal, 77, 79
temporal, 77, 79

Schwann cells, 28
Signs,
cerebellar, 30, 42, 54
Spinal border cells, 71
Spinal cord, 2-21, 59
Strabismus, 38
external, 54, 56
internal, 40
Subacute combined degeneration of the spinal cord, 12, 13
Substantia nigra, 60, 62, 74, 82, 83, 84, 85, 88-90, 92
lesions of, 84
Subthalamic nucleus,
lesion of, 88
Sulcus,
calcarine, 78-80
Swallowing and speech,
difficulty in, 26
Sweating,
diminution (or loss) of, 10
Sympathetic chain, 27
Syndrome,
Brown-Séquard, 2, 10
Claude's, 56
Déjérine-Roussy, 74
dorsal midbrain, 58
Horner's, 27, 40
lateral medullary, 26
medial medullary, 24, 25
medial pontine, 38, 39
Millard-Gubler, 46, 47
neocerebellar, 56
of jugular foramen, 32
Parinaud's, 58
thalamic, 74, 75, 90
Wallenberg's, 26, 34
Weber's 54, 55, 57
Wernicke's, 70
Syringohydromyelia, 6
Syringomyelia, 6-9, 18, 19
System,
anterolateral, 2-14, 16-18, 22, 23, 26, 27, 30, 34, 38-44, 46, 48, 50, 54, 56, 58-60, 62, 70, 75, 91, 93
dorsal column, 7, 22

Taste,
loss of, 28, 30
Temporal bone, 50
Thalamic nucleus(i), 86
anterior, 82, 88, 90, 92
centromedian (CM), 67, 82, 86-88, 90, 92
centromedian-parafascicular, 74
dorsomedial, 74, 82, 88, 90, 92
lateral dorsal, 88

parafascicular, 86, 87
pulvinar, 74
ventral anterior (VA), 67, 82, 88, 90
ventral lateral (VL), 67, 69, 74, 82, 86-88, 90, 92
ventral posterolateral (VPL), 7, 9, 11, 17, 23, 25, 27, 41, 43, 57, 74, 75, 82, 86, 88, 90-93
ventral posteromedial (VPM), 23, 41, 45, 57, 74, 82, 86, 88, 90-93
Thoracic cord injury, 16, 17
Tinnitus, 28
Titubation, 68, 70
Tongue, 24, 25, 28, 54, 55, 90
Tract(s), See also Fiber(s),
dorsal column, 22
dorsal spinocerebellar, 12, 71
lateral corticospinal, 2-4, 6, 8, 10-14, 16-18, 25, 39, 55, 67, 75, 83
lateral vestibulospinal, 69
mesencephalic, 54
optic, 59, 76-82, 90
rubrospinal, 12, 67
solitary, 22, 24, 26, 28, 30-32, 34, 35, 50
spinal trigeminal, 22-24, 26-28, 31, 32, 34, 35, 42-45, 48, 50
spinocerebellar, 6, 8, 14, 26
ventral spinocerebellar, 12, 71
Tremor, 68, 84
Truncal instability, 70
Tumor(s), 3
extramedullary, 2, 10
on dorsal roots, 2

Uncus,
herniation of, 62
Upward gaze.
loss of, 58, 78
Uvula, 55

Ventral root, 2, 4, 5, 9, 15
Ventricle,
fourth, 6
Vertebra(ae),
fracture, 16
Vertebral column, 4, 16
Vertigo, 28
Visual cortex,
lesion of, 78
Visual field,
nasal, 77, 79
temporal, 77, 79
Vomiting, 58, 62
Zona incerta, 82, 86, 88, 92
Zone of Lissauer, 6, 10, 16, 17